RESEARCH GUIDELINES:
A HANDBOOK FOR THERAPISTS

£7. 95

Fiona Collen
Feb. 1988.
Rivermead
OXFORD

Research Guidelines: A Handbook for Therapists

Cecily J Partridge FCSP BA PhD
Rosemary E Barnitt Dip COT BSc MSc

Heinemann Physiotherapy
London

First published in 1986 by
William Heinemann Medical Books, 23 Bedford Square,
London WC1B 3HH

0 433 24710 X

Typeset by Latimer Trend, Plymouth and
printed in Great Britain by Biddles
Limited, Guildford

Preface

We had therapists in mind when preparing these guidelines for research, but they could be useful to any clinician who wants to undertake their own study or evaluate published research material.

Editorials and leading articles in national professional journals have for some years been exhorting their members to evaluate their practice critically by becoming involved in research. While this is a possible option for an increasing number of health care professionals who have followed degree courses, there are still many practising clinicians who do not have direct access to research resources and lack basic research skills; this book should help them.

We have used the material in this book for work with students; we have also found that more experienced researchers find it helpful as a reference when actually setting up a project. It is based on the workshops and seminars on research we have organised over the past eight years, and we are most grateful to all who attended them for making us realise that a book like this was needed and for never accepting easy answers.

Cecily Partridge
Rosemary Barnitt

Contents

1 Stages of the Research Process

Since undertaking any investigation means becoming involved in a process of research this is the central focus of the book. Research is a scientific process, and there is a sequence that must be followed, a series of stages each based on the work of earlier stages. A large part of the work in any investigation is done before the collection of information actually begins, and starting to collect your 'facts' before sufficient planning has been undertaken is dangerous. It is the calibre of the preliminary work which sets the standard for the whole project, and the effect of skimping or hurrying in the early stages leaves its mark on the rest of the work. Studies which are not carefully planned rarely provide useful information.

This book is based on the concept of research as a scientific process and, however small or large your study, most of the following stages will have to be considered in the sequence given. There is a brief summary of the stages and a checklist (see p.4) only in this chapter, as the following chapters expand these aspects in more detail.

Stage 1

This starts with asking questions and developing ideas.

1 This may be questioning some aspect of practice, leading to other ideas, which usually raise further questions. Write them down and try them out on other people.
2 Reading the literature is essential to try to find out if other people have had the same ideas, also to see the type of investigations that have been undertaken in your area of interest and the results reported. Reading around your topic also helps to fill in the general background.
3 Defining the research question comes next and is usually

a difficult task; to be successful it must be clear, concise and unambiguous. As this question forms the basis of the whole project, its importance cannot be overstressed.

4 When you are satisfied that your question is clearly defined a statement of the objectives of the study or the hypotheses proposed must be given. Exact and clear statements are needed here as they were for the research question.

Stage 2

Deciding on the appropriate research design—this must fit the question and the objectives—not the other way round. A poor starting point is 'let's do a survey'.

1 Organising approaches to the fieldwork comes next. This involves a good deal of personal contact and much planning to ensure that nothing is missed out that can jeopardise the project.

2 Writing the research proposal is much easier if the preparatory work has been well done but, nevertheless, it takes time.

3 If you are going to apply for funding, this is the stage at which to apply to grant-awarding bodies. Fieldwork involves finding out the particular interest of different funding bodies so that adequate information about the proposed work can be given, highlighting relevant points for each organisation.

4 Ethical committees and other bodies concerned with the use of human subjects in research must not be forgotten—their permission may have to be obtained before starting the work. They will usually want to see the research proposal and will probably require additional information about ethical issues such as safety and confidentiality.

Stage 3

Now you are ready to consider methods of collecting information and to prepare forms and questionnaires.

1 This will involve considering the validity and reliability of the tests to be used and possibly developing and testing tools specifically for the project.
2 Consideration needs to be given to how the data collected will be analysed; discussion with others will probably be necessary. Decisions about whether a computer will be needed for the analysis may affect the ways in which you collect your data. Consultation with a statistician may be a good idea at this point.

Stage 4

This stage is concerned with actually collecting the information, and the stage most people have been waiting for.

1 First, you must run a pilot study where you test out the methods you are going to use—the dummy run—which is an essential part of the process.
2 When any necessary adjustments have been made, the main study can start—this is where the value of all the early work becomes clear. Things will go much more smoothly if time and care have been spent on preceding stages.

Stage 5

When all the information is collected you are now in the final stages of the work.

1 Analysis of results is undertaken using methods planned in Stage 3.
2 The report is written up including all the work from your original ideas, through the literature and planning stages down to the results which must be interpreted and discussed in relation to the research question.
3 Finally the results are presented in both written and verbal forms—no one is going to know about your work unless you tell them!

Although these stages should be considered in sequence it will often be necessary to pass backwards and forwards between the stages while you are undertaking your study.

	Yes	No	Not applicable
1 Asking questions, developing ideas			
Reading the literature			
Defining the research question			
Statement of objectives for the study, or producing a hypothesis for testing			
2 Deciding on appropriate research design			
Organisation and approaches to field work			
Writing the research proposal			
Applying to grant-awarding bodies			
Ethical committees or other bodies concerned with the use of human subjects			
3 Considering methods of collecting information			
Preparing forms and questionnaires			
Considering analysis of data			
Consulting a statistician			
4 Collection of information			
Pilot work			
Main study			
5 Analysis of results			
Writing the report			
Presentation of oral and written papers			

Fig. 1.1 *Checklist.*

2 Developing Ideas and Defining the Research Question

The goal of research in clinical practice is to find the answer to a problem using scientific procedures. Applied research should always start from problems encountered in practice. The selection of the topic will be dependent on the researcher's own experience and feelings about what is interesting and important.

A therapist working with patients with head injuries saw an article written by a consultant neurologist in which the value of rehabilitation with these patients was queried. In particular, it was stated that there would be little functional recovery after three months post injury. The therapist felt strongly, in the light of her own experience of treating patients with head injuries, that this assumption was wrong and set up a research project to investigate longer term progress with patients receiving physical therapy. The results showed that even two years post injury some patients were still achieving functional improvement. As this example shows, there will usually be some personal involvement and commitment to the research; this helps to maintain enthusiasm and interest when dealing with the problems and the more boring routine work which is part of any research. However, to reduce any subjective bias due to clinical enthusiasm, it is essential to demonstrate that objective scientific methods have been used.

Ideas and problems identified for research seldom come from neat intellectual exercises carried out by the researcher. In the main they stem from doubts the clinician has about the treatment procedures being used, articles they have read, comments made by patients or fellow workers; any of which can lead to a feeling of uncertainty and wanting to find out more. Journal articles and textbooks often give confident statements about events which, on reflection, are quite unsubstantiated. One which has appeared in medical textbooks for the past 40 years is that people with multiple sclerosis have periods when they demonstrate a 'euphoric' mood, but no evidence is given.

A researcher held strong views about the benefits of one walking aid over several others available to arthritic patients. By selecting a sample of patients from two other departments as well as her own, and by videoing the patient's walking ability, and asking independent assessors to rate this, she controlled any bias which could have been due to her own enthusiasm for the particular aid she favoured. Results from independent assessors are demonstrably unbiased.

Books on how to do research and many research articles, start with a description of the topic followed by the aims of carrying out the research. There is seldom any indication of how the researcher managed to define the problem in the first place. Clinicians who have started to do research without guidance have found that this first stage in the process can be quite difficult. The cycle of events which most researchers pass through is shown below.

1 Getting an idea
    ↓
2 Thinking through the idea
    ↓
3 Checking the idea against the literature and discussion with other people
    ↓
4 Defining the research question
    ↓
5 Setting specific research aims, objectives or hypotheses

1   Getting an idea

Ideas for research in clinical practice come from three principal sources.

Policy problems

The first of these is in relation to policy problems. Policy makers in central government and local management teams are concerned with providing a service to patients. The information which they want from research concerns numbers and needs. How many physiotherapists do we need in a day hospital serving 40 patients? How many occupational therapists are needed in social service departments to fulfil the statutory requirements for the provision of services. How many family practitioners are needed for each 100 000 people in the population?

Underlying these management and policy problems are more complex practical issues. There is little point in asking how many therapists are needed to help the disabled person without also looking at ways of preventing disability arising in the first place; research on preventive practice is still in its infancy in the therapy field.

Existing research

The second source of research ideas is existing research. It is quite common to pick up a research article and see in the discussion section suggestions for 'further' work which needs carrying out, as in the example given below.

> 'The findings of the study provide material for several subsequent studies, for example, to investigate why so many people attending the day hospital in the rural area had need of social support, why several people had been attending for over a year, and whether those attending for nursing procedures only would have been as well treated by a community nurse.'
>
> A. Cousins and S. Hale
> A comparative study of referrals and the work undertaken at two geriatric day hospitals. In *Rehabilitation—Selected Papers*, Kings Fund Centre (1983)

This second example also gives ideas for further research which have been generated by a completed study.

'Several advantages could accrue from a greater emphasis on home care and rehabilitation for stroke patients:

1 The rehabilitation given can be more closely tailored to the patient's needs and expectations.
2 Anxiety and depression may well be reduced in both the patient and his relatives.
3 There might be more effective use of limited resources. Fewer patients would need to be admitted, and those admitted might be able to be discharged home sooner.

At present these ideas are unproven. There is a great need for research into health care policies including the appropriate relation between home and hospital care.'

D. T. Wade and R. L. Hewer
Why admit stroke patients to hospital? *The Lancet*, 9 April (1983), pp. 807–808

Evaluation of practice

The third source of research ideas relates to the relative youth of the professions allied to medicine. In the past decade the number of procedures used by therapists and others has increased dramatically. Many of these skills and techniques have received little, if any, evaluation of their use and efficacy in relation to patient care.

The following questions are often asked:

When is it most appropriate to see the patient, straight after injury, at the start of the illness, or is there a critical time lapse?
Where is it best to give therapy, in the ward, in the department, in the patient's own home, or elsewhere?
Which methods of therapy are most effective with different conditions?
How frequently should treatment be given, every hour or once a week?
How long should the treatment last? How should the patient be positioned?
Why should treatment be given at all, does it make any difference to the patient's progress or recovery?

Ideas are plentiful, the next stage is to know what to do with an idea which you want to develop further.

2 Thinking through the idea

An idea selected for research should be simple, the topic should be important to the potential researcher, and finally the possible outcome should have clear implications for change to the benefit of the patient or the service. There is little point, and much disappointment, in completing a demanding piece of research and finding that the only recommendations possible from it are 'more money' or 'more staff'. Thinking through the possible outcome of an investigation is an extremely important part of early work.

Ideas for research often start with a general, diffuse, and possibly confused notion of what the problem is; the problem, therefore, has to be ordered into shape, so that research questions can be formulated. This is illustrated in the following example.

A number of occupational therapists have been interested in carrying out research to find out more about the efficacy of the aids which they issue to patients. If one of these researchers decided that the research area was 'aids', this could mean looking at over 5000 items of equipment. Even if the decision was to limit the topic by looking at aids in relation to patients with rheumatoid arthritis (RA) this could still involve many hundreds of aids. The wise researcher may well settle for researching 'cutlery for RA patients'. If this is the case, would the study still reflect the original idea of the efficacy of aids?

The researcher who is thinking widely will find that he comes up with a variety of topics, and then picks the one that is most interesting to him. Staying with the idea of aids, this could generate several studies: 'design of aids', 'access and supply of aids', 'cost of aids', 'training in use of aids', and others. The original idea has now given rise to many possible research topics.

It is wise to realise that although a large topic area may seem potentially of much greater interest, experienced researchers know that the only hope of obtaining any worthwhile result is to concentrate initially on a small, clearly defined topic. There are a number of different techniques used to help in arriving at an appropriate topic. Two methods are briefly described.

Brain storming

Write the idea or problem at the top of a sheet of paper and then list underneath it any word or phrase which you think is associated with it. It is often useful to get other people to help with this. Once all the words have been listed the main theme can be sorted out under category headings. The following is an example, starting from the topic of patients who have had an amputation.

Idea

Amputees and their problems

Contractures	Crutches	Housing
Wheelchair	Pressure sores	Family
Diabetes	Limb fitting	Occupation
Elderly	Stump bandaging	Mobility
Visual problems	Emotional state	Shock
Adjustment	Stigma	Sex

Categories

Psychological	*Physical*	*Social*
Stigma	Diabetes	Family
Adjustment	Contractures	Housing
Emotional state	Elderly	Occupation
Shock	Visual problems	
Sex	Crutches	
Phantom limb	Limb fitting	
	Stump bandaging	
	Sex	
	Wheelchair	
	Pressure sores	
	Mobility	

Research topics stemming from this could include: 'Amputees and housing problems'; 'Amputees and emotional adjustment'; 'Contractures following amputation'; 'Stump bandaging and the phantom limb'. There are almost endless permutations starting from a single topic.

Pattern notes

This technique is described by Tony Buzan in *Use Your Head* (1982). He suggests that making notes in straight lines across and down the page is alien to the way many people think. He advocates starting with the topic in the centre of the sheet of paper and developing ideas along lines or dividing branches as is shown in Fig. 2.1.

Research topics stemming from this could be the 'Community physiotherapists' relationship with family prac-

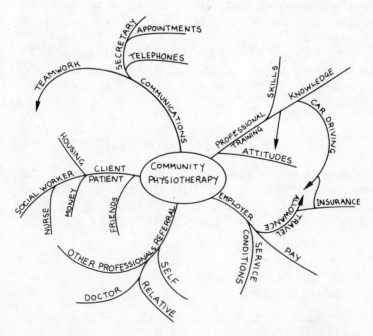

Fig. 2.1   *Pattern notes.*

titioners, neighbours, or relatives'. Or, the 'Therapist's access to transport or telephones'. As with brain storming such a plan suggests many research topics.

3   Checking the idea against the literature and discussion with other people

Once the idea has been expanded and a particular aspect of the problem selected, it is important to check to see if other researchers are asking questions in your area of interest and, if so, where your own research problem fits in. This involves carrying out a literature search (*see* Chapter 3 for further details). Only by examining what other people have done and are thinking about in your particular area can your idea be fitted into the right context. Is it a controversial topic, is there general agreement in the area, what have other people found?

Discussing your ideas with other people is equally important. Try explaining your idea to a friend or colleague then get them to explain back to you what you have been saying. This will tell you how clearly you are thinking! Do not only discuss it with friends; critical comment is very helpful in sharpening your defence of the idea—if it is defensible.

4   Defining the research question

When you are satisfied that the early thinking stage has been fully explored and you have emerged with an interesting problem you wish to research, the next stage is to define the research question. What is most important is that it is:

1 Clear and unambiguous.
2 Answerable within the resources available—these include time, finance and skills.
3 Practical in application.

The question may be concerned with relationships between different topics. For example:

Does speech therapy education lead to a knowledge of psycho-linguistic theory?
Do patients with non-specific lumbar pain benefit from manipulation techniques?
Can play therapy help young disturbed children?
Does the nursing process promote good care for the elderly?

Absolutely clear definitions of all the words in the proposed question are needed. If a word or expression cannot be defined it cannot be researched. From the specified: speech therapy education, psycholinguistic theory, non-specific lumbar pain, manipulation techniques, play therapy, young disturbed children, the nursing process, good care, and the elderly. Taking what may seem the most obvious one from that list, the elderly, it may be assumed that everyone knows who the elderly are. In research terms it could mean women over 60 and men over 65, which are the official pensionable and retirement ages in Britain; both men and women over 65, over 70, or perhaps even over 75.

Getting these terms correct once again is a lengthy process. After considerable effort you may come up with a question that is clear and unambiguous but may not now represent your original purpose. In this case it is back to the drawing board.

The necessity for a good question cannot be overstressed as without it you have little hope of a workable project.

In applied research it is not only important to have a good clear question but also to consider the practical uses to which the information can be put. Will there be a possibility of the results influencing practice such as improving some aspect of organisation, management, or care given to patients?

5   Setting specific research aims, objectives and hypotheses

The final stage in this defining process is to write down the general aim of the research, and specific objectives which are to be achieved. The following example illustrates the specificity needed in stating objectives, which can then be used as the basis for the investigation.

In a study of community physiotherapy which had the broad aim of describing a sample of community physiotherapy services, the following specific objectives were agreed after considerable discussion. The area was very diverse and clear objectives were necessary.

1 To define those patients and their conditions that were being seen in:
   (a) their own homes or other places of permanent residence;
   (b) general practice premises (other than health centres);
   (c) health centres.
2 Those patients receiving treatment from private practitioners of physiotherapy were excluded from the study.
3 To find from the selected schemes the nature, duration and frequency of the physiotherapy measures the patients were receiving.
4 To examine the relationship of the physiotherapist to others in the community concerned with the immediate care of the patient.
5 To describe the referral, review and discharge procedures of the patient, the accessibility and source of medical advice, and the physiotherapists' opinions about the adequacy of these procedures.
6 To examine the physiotherapist's relationship to others working in the hospital and in the social services department.

Then if the evidence favoured the development of services outside hospital:

7 To consider the future organisation of such services and to estimate the resources required.
8 To outline tentative schemes of physiotherapy outside hospital, indicating priorities.
9 To make recommendations about future training for such a service.

In some circumstances, it is possible to go further than stating objectives by preparing and writing down an hypothesis or set of hypotheses which are to be tested during the research. An hypothesis is a conjectural statement of the relation between two or more variables (*see* Glossary for further definition).

The word 'guesstimate' may help in understanding the concept. An hypothesis is your 'guess' about what may happen or be happening in a particular situation. Beveridge's (1974) statement that 'the hypothesis is the most important mental technique of the investigator, and its main function is to suggest new experiments and new observations' emphasises the continuing nature of the formulation of hypotheses.

Finding evidence to support an hypothesis which the investigator has set up as the basis of a study can seem to be an all-important end in itself, but hypotheses should be used as tools to uncover new facts rather than as ends in themselves.

In many investigations where hypotheses turn out to be unsupported, as many do, further hypotheses are derived which extend the work in a useful way and contribute to knowledge in the area.

It is important to remember that even if the evidence does support your hypothesis, further experimental work is needed before confidence can be placed in your idea. Significant results can only be true for the particular circumstances in which the research took place unless the study fulfils the criteria of statistical generalisation (*see* Glossary for further definitions).

An hypothesis statement contains two or more variables that are measurable or potentially measurable and specifies how the variables are related.

Variables are identified in research by the function that they perform. Independent variables are those which will be manipulated in the study, dependent variables are those which vary as a result of this manipulation.

Consider a simple hypothesis:

> 'Early mobilisation following surgery contributes to earlier discharge of patients from hospital.'

We have here a relation between one independent variable, mobilisation, and another dependent variable, discharge from hospital. Since measurement of these variables appears possible, it is likely that this can be tested as an hypothesis.

Consider a second hypothesis:

> 'Practice in memory skills has no effect on future ability to carry out memory tasks.'

This hypothesis is given in the so-called 'null' form; it says that one variable will have no effect on another. This is one way of stating an hypothesis, and the purpose of the research would be to find out if this assumption is correct, or if practice in memory skills really does turn out to have an effect on memory tasks. However, there is another kind of difficulty with this second hypothesis, and this is in defining and measuring both memory skills and future ability. If the difficulties of definition and measurement can be overcome this hypothesis may be testable. Great specificity is required in composing an hypothesis, both in selecting and defining the variables and in identifying the nature of the relationship between them.

In clinical practice there are not many research problems which can be defined in the form of these highly specific hypotheses. The clinical researcher will often find that he is dealing with aims and objectives. This does not mean that the research is not as good, rather that the researcher has selected the approach which is suitable for investigating the particular problem. The procedure for arriving at either an hypothesis or a set of objectives requires time and clear thinking. Throughout the definition process the overall aims of the investigation must be kept in mind.

Only when the research question, the aims and objectives of the research, and possibly the hypotheses, are clearly defined and written down can the design and methods for carrying out the research be considered. It may be tempting to decide to 'do a survey' before defining the research question, but the research question must decide the design or methods to be used and not the other way round. Before going on to discuss these research designs in Chapter 4, details of how to undertake a literature search are given in the next chapter.

References

Beveridge W. I. B. (1974). *The Art of Scientific Investigation.* London: Heinemann Educational Books.

Buzan T. (1982). *Use Your Head.* London: Ariel Books, BBC.

3 Searching the Literature

Closely following on from defining the research question is finding out what has already been written about your chosen topic. There may be very little, but even if you cannot find any references at all it is very important to have undertaken a careful search so that you can set the scene for your study and state in the introduction to your research proposal that 'few references to work in this area were found'. Beware of saying 'no references were found' even if *you* found none—someone else is sure to find at least one!

There are often strong generally held impressions about various areas of practice—things you 'know' that would be generally agreed by most clinicians—these alone cannot form the basis for any study, although they are a very useful starting point.

It is important not only to read about the topic that you are actually investigating but also to read round the subject, this provides the background and puts your study into perspective. For example, if you are interested in elderly patients with osteoarthrosis, not only should the obvious topics of the elderly and osteoarthrosis be pursued, but it would be wise to read about studies of other arthropathies and other knee conditions in both older and younger patients.

A study planned to examine the effect of relaxation classes for depressed patients would involve wide reading, including types of techniques used in relaxation, different manifestations of depression and the place of various types of exercise and relaxation for different types of psychiatric patients.

The aim of the literature search in the first place is to provide you with a list of references to articles and books in your chosen area. There may be a great many, in which case you will want to select those you are going to read, or only a few when you will probably want to read them all.

The basic steps in a search are set down below in a series of stages that can either be used as a checklist if you are having problems finding literature or as guidelines if you have not carried out this type of search before.

1 Select the aspects that you are interested in around your chosen topic and try to find *key* words. These are not always obvious and easy to decide—if you can find an article to start with in your area that has key words on it this could start you off, otherwise experiment. Librarians will be happy to try one or two out for you. A few examples from different journals may help:

Amputation as a consequence of diabetes mellitus: an epidemiological review.
Key words: Amputation—Diabetes mellitus—Epidemiology

Physical therapy for children with chronic lung disease.
Key words: Respiratory disease—Paediatrics—Physical therapy

Trends in clinical practice—an analysis of competencies.
Key words: Curriculum—Competencies—Education

Parents and therapists in a professional partnership.
Key words: Child development—Handicap—Occupational therapy—Professional patient relations

---

If the key words you give the librarian fail to retrieve the type of references you want, find others and try again. There is nothing magic about key words, they are just words that describe the content of the article. Titles may be misleading which means you may sometimes get inappropriate references from a key word.

2 Choosing a library is the next step and it is important to find one with a good librarian, one who gets satisfaction from helping you to get what you want, so if you are not lucky the first time try to find another. You may also

want to use different libraries for different purposes. The usual centres where books and journals on medical and allied subjects are held are postgraduate medical centres, training institutions of health care professions, universities and other institutes of higher education.

Many more libraries are available in large centres and some will keep information about where journals they do not hold are available. Do not hesitate to ask for help, one of the main functions of a library is to provide information.

Some libraries put together selected abstracts on different topic areas which could start you off if they have one that includes your particular area of interest.

When you have your key words noted down, select an appropriate library and try to be specific about what you want. It is irritating for the librarian to be asked for 'all necessary references' on a particular topic! Remember you can start with one aspect of your work and expand later as you begin to be familiar with the library system, but searching always takes longer than anticipated.

Librarians can help in locating the journals and will show you how to use the library indexing system. *Index Medicus*, which lists all articles related to medical topics published in most learned journals throughout the world, is a monthly publication held by most medical libraries and is also available in bound yearly editions. *The Science Citation Index* is a similar system for non-medical scientific articles.

You may be advised to run a computer search on your chosen topic, and here a system called *Medline* is sometimes recommended. At the start it is a good idea to do some hand searching yourself to get a feel for references in your chosen field and begin to recognise some of the writers in your area who have either written many articles or who are referred to frequently by others.

3 How far back to search is often a problem. If it is a popular topic with a large number of references, perhaps five years is reasonable to start with, but if references are scarce it may be worth going back 20 or even 30 years.

There are sometimes very early key references which are important.

4 Having obtained your list of references you will want some of the articles. Libraries often impose a limit of six or eight but this gives you a chance to go through the first batch and select later ones from your list more carefully as you become more familiar with the particular area.

Remember that each article will also have a list of references at the end and so it is very important to keep your particular topic and key words in mind, so that you strike the right balance between following all interesting lines of thought—in which case you may get far too many references and disappear beneath mountains of paper—and following your original key words too narrowly, which could mean that you miss some important work.

When you read the papers, if you find one or two articles are frequently referred to, it is wise to read them, even if they are 30 years old—they are obviously influential in the field.

Keeping the references

If you are undertaking a project of any kind, start a reference system straight away. Small cards are probably best, marked clearly with all details necessary to obtain the articles; you might wish to give the details to someone else, or even lose or mislay the paper. For a journal article, record the full names and initials of all authors, the title of the paper, the full name of the journal, the year, the volume number and the page numbers. For a book, record the title, the date, the publishers and place of publication. For a section within a book in addition give the editors of the book.

The articles can be filed alphabetically by author, and the cards filed according to the topic—where more than one topic is covered it is possible to cross-reference and have more than one card in different sections for the same article.

Other systems can be used but make sure you do have a system that serves your needs and that is clear and easy to use. It is relatively simple to start at the beginning of a project with only a few references, but very difficult indeed when you have accumulated a large number. If you are working on a project or have a continuing interest in a topic it may be worth telling your librarian, some will be prepared to contact you when new references come up in your areas of interest.

It is not enough to have read the articles and referenced them, it is also necessary to write a critical review of the articles you have collected and to summarise the important aspects. This review can be part of your final report or of itself can sometimes be suitable for publication.

When this is completed consideration can be given to finding an appropriate research design for the study.

4 Research Design

I Selection

'Most authors write as if they are the first to explore their subjects. They fail to take advantage of previous investigators ... There are many rewards to be derived from consulting the maps of previous explorers, even though these charts require correction and redrawing.' (Alpert, 1963, quoted by Easthope, 1974.)

In undertaking research, therapists will find that there are a number of research designs already available to them. Some of them will have been identified during the literature search. Whenever possible, a design should be selected that has been tried and tested in previous research. As Easthope says, advantage should always be taken of earlier developmental work. The design is the plan or scheme that will be used in the investigation and it is therefore important that the appropriate design for the proposed research is selected.

Research in the clinical field often cannot use the methodology of the natural sciences. This is because the material to be studied is fundamentally different from that of the natural scientist; human subjects cannot be studied or investigated in the same way as rock crystals or atoms. In practical terms this means that the people acting as subjects in clinical research may, at times, refuse to cooperate, have visitors when you want to interview them or die when you are halfway through the study! Some of the poorest clinical research has resulted from the selection of a design intended to study the phenomena of natural science instead of selecting a design suitable for studying human beings.

In selecting a research design the clinician first needs to answer the following questions.

1   Can I cope with this design? Do I have the skills and knowledge necessary for this type of study?

If the answer is no or you are not sure, it is best to consult others such as statisticians, physiological technicians, epidemiologists or computer scientists. The researcher has to be realistic about the time it will take to do the research, and the number of subjects that can be recruited to the sample. Data collection, interviewing, and data analysis can be unpredictable and time consuming. Computers have a habit of breaking down just when you are completing the final analysis of the data, and ambulances can be off the road on some of the days you have set up treatment sessions.

Experienced clinical researchers are familiar with the frustration of the 'disappearing' diagnosis. Under these conditions the researcher aims to include in the sample the first 50 new admissions to a particular hospital with diagnoses of, say, cerebrovascular accident, amputation, or multiple sclerosis. After two years the researcher is still waiting to complete the sample! Because these diagnostic groups have high dependence needs there is a tendency for clinicians to overestimate how many patients are available in their departments over a specific time period. The assumption had been made that many patients with a specific condition would be available, rather than checking with records.

Having found a sample, the researcher then has to plan how long the research will take. If a group of patients is to be followed up for one year after treatment, the research will have to continue until the last subject admitted to the sample has been discharged for one year; this probably means a three-year study. Finally, the clinical researcher needs to consider the cost of the research using the proposed design. Costs and funding are considered in depth in Chapter 5.

2 Can my subjects and colleagues cope with this design?

Research is never carried out in isolation, it requires the goodwill and cooperation of many people. Colleagues can become weary and eventually antagonistic to research which impinges too much on their job. For example, a research design used with the selected patient group may have a time-of-day effect, patients with rheumatoid arthritis may need to be tested on physical activity at the same time of day depending on patterns of pain and stiffness. Elderly patients may be mentally more alert in the morning than the afternoon. This means that the researcher may want priority in seeing certain patients in certain places at certain times of day. Nurses, porters, other therapists and relatives may, at times, be inconvenienced and therefore the design that interferes least with routine work should be selected.

Subjects who are physically or mentally unwell can find research procedures tiring and sometimes upsetting. If a questionnaire is to be used, remember that questions about home and family life can be distressing for a patient who is worried about their relationships because of their illness. One patient with multiple sclerosis expressed his appreciation to the researcher that during an interview he had been able to unburden his fears about his future life with his wife and family. Both researcher and patient became involved and when the time came to finish the interview the patient was so exhausted he fell out of his wheelchair!

Subjects can be placed in awkward situations if the research requires skills which they find difficult or impossible. It is hard for many people to admit that they cannot read or write and, therefore, cannot follow written instructions. Elderly subjects often do not admit, even to themselves, that hearing and vision are failing. Patients with speech disorders may be upset if they are not included in research because they are difficult to understand. Tact and tolerance must be exhibited by the researcher in ensuring that participants in the research feel comfortable, and realise that their contribution is of value.

3 Is the design appropriate and ethical?

A good deal of nonsense is talked about the status of research designs. It is often suggested that designs that mimic most closely those of natural science are 'best', and that social science models are not as good. This is not true; the best design is the one which suits the research question. In medicine particularly, the double-blind controlled trial has been seen as an ideal design. In this design, which was originally intended to test the effect of drugs, a number of subjects are selected and divided into two or more groups. One of these groups receives the active treatment, while the other, the control group, receives no active treatment, only a placebo. The design ensures that neither the person administering the treatment nor the person receiving it knows which is the active treatment and which the placebo. In this way it is possible to find out the effects of a drug without bias.

However, in many clinical situations where treatment cannot be delivered in measured doses of medication in the form of tablets and where replica pills cannot be used as placebos, other research designs are more appropriate, and these will be discussed in the second part of this chapter.

II Examples

Five types of research design most frequently used by clinicians are briefly described in this chapter. There are, however, many more in the research literature and these can be found in the books given in the Bibliography.

1 Retrospective studies

It may be possible to answer the research question by reference to an existing database (see, for example, box opposite).

One of the problems of relying on existing records is that some essential information may be missing as records kept for treatment and other department purposes may not be in a suitable form for the study.

How many women over the age of 65 attend accident and emergency departments as a result of a fall in the home?

This information may be available from casualty records and patient case notes.

Are more patients with chest conditions referred to a physiotherapy department between December and March than between April and July?

This information may be found in physiotherapy records.

Filing systems may be based on the patient's name, or a particular doctor's clinic, which means that you cannot retrieve the information you need according to age or diagnostic category. Sometimes it is possible to set up a recording system so that in the future the data can be used for study purposes. Some departments code patients according to their ICD code (the International Classification of Diseases, 1969). When this is done notes can be recalled on the basis of diagnostic category as each disease or condition is categorised by a number within the ICD.

2 Descriptive studies

When carried out systematically and rigorously, descriptive studies can be a valuable source of information. Historically, research has always started with observation and description. Harvey, who discovered the mechanisms of the circulatory system in the sixteenth century, meticulously observed and described the functioning of the arteries and veins and the cardiac system. Description is an essential stage in establishing a professional knowledge base. Descriptive studies can be undertaken of patient groups, the use of a piece of equipment or some aspect of service provision including treatment techniques. Some examples of descriptive studies are given below.

The first example shows how a study which describes the follow-up of a group of diabetic patients gives valuable information about future service needs.

Example The Diabetic, the Hospital and Primary Care

E. Wilkes and E. E. Lawton
Journal of Royal College of General Practitioners, April 1980, p. 199

SUMMARY. In a survey of mainly elderly patients discharged from a hospital diabetic clinic, it was found that 41% were being seen by the general practitioner only when required or not at all, 36% were being seen fairly regularly, and 23% at routine appointments.

The transfer from hospital to primary care was popular with two-thirds of these patients, mainly because of the time, trouble, and money they saved in no longer travelling to hospital.

Over 20% of patients thought they had been discharged from the diabetic clinic because they were cured, a further 37% thought they could be cured, about a third did not test their urine, and a similar proportion admitted that they did not keep to their diet.

Of 204 known diabetics examined in general practice, about half had high blood sugars, a third of lower limbs had undoubted signs of peripheral vascular disease, and one fifth of the sample had both. This example shows that by following up a group of patients valuable information can be gained about service and delivery.

The second example demonstrates how it is possible to achieve a number of aims by describing a service accurately.

Example Referrals to an Occupational Therapy Division:
A Descriptive Survey

W. Smart, M. Vaughan, S. Hunt
Occupational Therapy, March 1983, pp. 83–85

The specific objective was to make a descriptive survey of the Occupational Therapy Section of the Nottingham Social Services Department, identifying the basic characteristics of the service and providing much needed information in the following areas: main source of referral, length of waiting time between referral and evaluation, age and sex distribution of clients, disability assessment, diagnosis, and types of aids and adaptations recommended.

Some therapists are concerned that research will discredit the work they do. No service is perfect and having more information will identify ways in which the service can be improved. This is well illustrated by this third example.

Example   An Investigation into the Management of Bilateral Leg Amputees

C. Van de Ven
British Medical Journal, 1981, 283, 707–710

Patients with bilateral high level amputations of the legs are rarely functionally independent after their discharge from hospital. Eighty bilateral amputees were visited by a research physiotherapist, and information was obtained on their family circumstances, accommodation, mobility and prostheses.

A second questionnaire was completed by hospital staff on medical condition, assessments, rehabilitation, and total overall management.

The results showed that mobility was severely restricted; out of the 80 patients visited, only 65 could manoeuvre wheelchairs and 23 used prostheses. Accommodation presented difficulties: 34 homes had steps inside and 40 had steps outside. Of the 80 patients seen, 60 could not cope in the bath while 33 were unable to use the lavatory. Assessments and rehabilitation were lacking. There appeared to be little overall management, and hospital staff made only 36 visits to the patients' accommodation before discharge.

Another example of the use of descriptive research is in the first stage of an evaluative study. There are very few 'standard' methods of treatment and management in remedial therapy, and a first stage before examining the efficacy of any treatment or management procedures is accurately describing them so that you and others can be sure of exactly what the treatment or management procedures were.

3 Clinical trials

Clinical trials are set up to test the efficacy of different methods of treatment. The clinical situation is controlled as far as is possible, and then the effect of the treatment is studied. Three types of design come under this heading: double blind, single blind and comparative studies.

Double-blind controlled trials

This design has already been described on page 26 with regard to medical drug trials. The essential characteristics of the design are that patients are allocated to either an 'active' or 'control' group and the treatment outcome for both groups is then compared. The criterion for this design is that *neither* patient *nor* staff administering treatment, *nor* the researchers assessing the results, know which patients have received the 'active' treatment. In this way bias is eliminated from the results, and if changes have occurred only in the 'active' group, they can be reliably attributed to the treatment given. This method is not often appropriate in remedial therapy as double-blind conditions can rarely be achieved; perhaps one of the few instances where it may be possible is with electrical treatments. With the use of a computer connected to the appliance and programmed for a random on/off series of treatments, while maintaining a standard display panel, the therapist can be unaware of whether an 'active' or 'inactive' treatment is being given.

Single-blind trials

The single-blind control design is similar in most respects to the double-blind design except that the clinician giving the treatment knows which treatment the patient is receiving. However, it is necessary to ensure that the assessor who is taking the measurements before and after treatment is blind to the allocation of patients to different groups. In one study a group of patients in long stay wards for the elderly were divided into groups and each group was given a different vitamin supplement. The idea was to see if certain vitamins improved mental awareness. A therapist was asked to carry out functional assessments on each patient at regular intervals, but did not know which vitamin supplement the patient had had. After a time, it was possible to compare the vitamins given with the functional improvement and see if there was a specific effect from any of them.

Comparative studies

In comparative research the purpose is to select two or

more treatments, conditions, or client groups so that similarities and differences can be studied. Often the subjects or groups to be compared are naturally occurring: for example, the comparison of referrals to two psychiatric day hospitals, the comparison of domiciliary physiotherapy services in different health districts, or the comparison of methods of teaching psycholinguistics to speech therapy students. Occasionally, the researcher will need to create the two groups for a comparative study; this is shown in the following example.

Example Recovery Trends of Functional Skills in the Head-Injured Adult

L. B. Panikoff
American Journal of Occupational Therapy, November 1983, 37, no. 11

This study describes the course of the recovery of functional skills in adults with severe head injuries during a two-year period. Eighty head-injured patients admitted to an inpatient rehabilitation unit were included in this study.

Length of coma could be ascertained for 78 of the patients. These subjects were then divided into two groups by coma length (i.e. less than or equal to 14 days coma and greater than or equal to 15 days coma) as defined by the Glasgow Coma Scale. All 80 patients were rated at 2-, 4-, 6-, 12-, and 24-month intervals after reported date of injury in the following areas: basic ADLs (feeding, grooming, bed mobility), wheelchair mobility, dressing, functional transfers, basic hand skills, community skills, kitchen skills, and Jebsen hand function.

An ethical problem sometimes arises, particularly in a double-blind trial, of some patients in the so-called 'control' group receiving no active treatment. According to strict ethical guidelines, this is quite acceptable, as you are only withholding a treatment whose value is unknown; if its value was known there would be no need to do the study. However, the clinicians actually administering the treatments often find this aspect particularly difficult. One way round the problem is to give all patients a basic standard treatment, then the active group receive the experimental treatment *in addition*. An example is given below:

A study to investigate the use of ultrasound to accelerate healing in strain to the lateral ligament of the ankle.

All subjects in Groups A and B receive:
   support bandage
   advice on elevation for swelling
   graduated exercise programme

Group A also receives, in addition, ultrasound insonation according to the agreed schedules.

---

4   Experimental or laboratory research designs

These are not used as frequently in remedial therapy as they are in some fields of psychology and the pure sciences. These studies are set up with the purpose of attempting to control as many sources of variability as possible. For an experimental study the naturally occurring situation is not examined. If you did want to carry out an experimental study in clinical practice you would expect to set up a special test area where items such as noise, light, heat, etc., could be strictly controlled, so that identical physical conditions for all subjects is ensured. You would also want to control for many other variables such as sex, age, marital status, diagnostic category, time of day and recency of intake of food and drink. In all research design, the aim is to control as many variables as is practical; however, in experimental studies it is imperative. The disadvantage of such stringent control is that patients and clients seldom perform in such conditions in real life so this design is useful for only a limited but important range of studies. A few examples may be helpful.

Reliability of Goniometric Measurements

D. C. Boone *et al.*
Physical Therapy, 1978, 58, 11, 1355–1359.

This study determined the intratester and intertester variability and reliability of goniometric measurements taken by four physical therapists of upper and lower extremity motions of normal male subjects.

The Effect of Pulsed Intrasound on Tissue Regeneration

M. Dyson and J. B. Pound
Physiotherapy, 1970, 56, 134–142

These experiments were carried out using the pinnae of rabbits' ears to compare tissue repair following injury in ears insonated with ultrasound as against those uninsonated.

When carrying out standardised tests there are usually comprehensive handbooks which indicate exactly how the test should be administered. The handbook is to help you to control a number of variables. The following example shows how such a test was standardised using an experimental approach.

Adult Norms for the Box and Block Test of Manual Dexterity

V. Mathiowetz *et al.*
American Journal of Occupational Therapy, June 1985, 386–391

The Box and Block Test, a test of manual dexterity, has been used by occupational therapists and others to evaluate physically handicapped individuals. Because the test lacked normative data for adults, the results of the test have been interpreted subjectively. The purpose of this study was to develop normative data for adults. Test subjects were 628 normal adults from the Milwaukee area. Data on males and females aged 20–94 years were divided into 12 age groups. Means, standard deviations, standard errors, and low and high scores were reported for each five-year age group. These data will enable clinicians to compare objectively a patient's score to that of a similar normal population.

5   Single case study designs

The single case study design method is often confused with the case study report and considered to be at an anecdotal level. However, as a research design, objective methods of measurement must be used and designs strictly followed.

This method has much to offer clinicians often as a first step towards evaluating and investigating different aspects of practice. The basis of the single case study design is to carry out repeated measurement of one subject. Classic single case study designs include the so-called ABA and ABAB. In these designs a baseline A performance is established of the aspect in which you are interested. An objective assessment of performance is undertaken using demonstrably reliable methods. The treatment you are investigating which has been clearly defined is given for a specified period of time, B, and then stopped when the baseline measurement A is repeated. Differences in the before and after measurements are examined. In the ABAB design, treatment is resumed, if effective, after the second baseline measurement. An example may help.

A client has problems of claustrophobia and cannot travel anywhere; he finds trains worse than cars. The baseline measurement *A* is the patient's anxiety ratings when attempting to travel by car and train or even when contemplating this.

B is the treatment, in this case progressive desensitisation and relaxation techniques, which are used for a two-week period.

A: One week after treatment has stopped anxiety ratings are taken again and reports of attempts at travelling taken. This is basically the ABA design. The ABAB design would be if the treatment *B* was again introduced.

The reader is referred to Herson and Barlow (1976) for an introduction to the subject.

References

Easthope G. (1974). *History of Social Research Methods.* London: Longman.

Herson M., Barlow D. H. (1976). *Single Case Experimental Design.* Oxford: Pergamon Press.

International Classification of Diseases (1969). Geneva: WHO.

5 Writing Research Proposals and Applying for Funds

1 Writing research proposals

Most funding bodies, universities and institutions of higher education provide their own forms that must be completed when applying for a research grant, but the common core of information that will be needed can be collected and then abstracted to put on the different application forms. You may often have to apply to more than one funding body, but it is usually wise to apply to only one at a time. Even if you are not putting in a formal application for funding, sorting out this information at the beginning will help clear thinking and organisation of the whole project. The research proposal may also be called a research protocol, but in practice the terms are used interchangeably.

The title

A short descriptive title is needed, not too long but giving sufficient information. An example may help.

An investigation into the use of bath aids and walking aids by patients over the age of 65 in the six-month period following their discharge from a small community hospital.
Too long

An investigation of the use of aids.
Too short

An investigation of the use of aids by elderly patients following discharge from hospital.
About right

The title should sound interesting and relate to an

important topic; if it is boring or unclear you will start off at a disadvantage.

Introduction

This should contain a brief summary of the problem you propose to study, with a few relevant references to previous work, or work in related areas. It is helpful to spell out clearly the questions which you think are important. Make this section as interesting as you can to persuade the reader at the outset of the worth of the project. You are setting the scene here for the rest of the proposal. Your job is to demonstrate logically but imaginatively that there is a gap in knowledge to be filled and then to explain how your study will contribute towards filling that gap. Clearly define the research question and any hypotheses (*see* Chapter 2) you are proposing.

Methods

This section must be explicit. It should contain sufficient detail to allow the reader to understand exactly how you propose to carry out the study. If this is your first proposal seek advice and study other successful proposals. It requires considerable judgement to know how much to include, and application forms only offer limited space. If methods you are going to use are well known a single reference to a published paper will suffice, but if new methods are to be used or developed they should be described in some detail in your formal application—if rather long or complex it may be more convenient to put them in an appendix with a statement in this section to that effect. Details of the subjects you propose to include, criteria for inclusion, exclusion, and methods of selection must be given. The data that will be collected must be described and methods of analysis and data processing briefly mentioned.

Successful applications are those which not only contain a well defined problem in the introduction but also a well defined approach in this methods section. You need to show here that not only have you asked a good question but also that you know how to investigate it. Detail here is not only important for the grant application but to be used as a reference throughout the study. Once you have started the main study things cannot be changed.

Facilities available

These must be described accurately. If equipment is required state whether it will be available within your work area or if it has to be purchased, or perhaps it might be available on loan.

It is essential to mention the names of other specialists in different fields who have agreed to be available for consultation or technical help. Other clinicians may help too but it is wise to ensure that academic help/advice is also available—if possible someone experienced in research. Do remember not to put anyone's name down unless you have their permission in writing. Copies of these letters may be included in a formal application.

Where the work will actually be carried out

This may be on one, or a number of sites. It is necessary here to name the institutions, and state that agreement has been obtained from them and from anyone whose permission is needed; here again written permission is advisable. Grant-awarding bodies will want to know who will be responsible for holding the research grant; this might be a hospital, medical faculty or academic institution. Written permission is a good idea even if a formal application is not being made. Confirming verbal agreements by letter is another safeguard. Staff change and by the time you come to do your project, the person you spoke to and who gave you permission may have left and without a letter no evidence of their agreement will be available.

Finances

It is often very difficult to calculate the cost of a project but you must arrive at a realistic estimate which will enable you to complete the job, here again consult others. Remember, in research, everything always takes much longer than you think; in Britain many projects are for three years, few less than two. You will have to work out not only the capital costs for any equipment you need but recurrent costs which should include the following:

1 Staff salaries, this to include health insurance, pension funds and other usual deductions.
2 Travel and subsistence.
3 Stationery and photocopying.
4 Postage and telephone.
5 Secretarial assistance.
6 Attendance at conferences.

Remember to allow for salary increases, and possible increases in post, telephone and other charges over the period of the study.

If you are only planning a small project and not applying for funding, it is still worth going through the process of considering your project under these headings, you may find when you have worked it all out that you do need some funding after all!

If you are applying for funding your proposal may have to go to a number of different bodies, but it is worth giving time when you are preparing your proposal to scrutinise the literature that comes with the application forms. Different funding bodies will have different interests. For research councils the emphasis will be on scientific method; charitable bodies will want to know how your research is related to their interests; whereas ethical committees will want to know how you are safeguarding the patients' interests.

It is a good idea to photocopy application forms and have a trial run before you finally complete them. It may be worth reiterating here how important it is to make a good impression. A clear typed copy is essential, clear presentation will increase your chance of success.

Curriculum vitae

Information about the person applying for a grant will be needed with previous publications listed if there are any. You want to give information here that demonstrates that you not only have a good research question and appropriate scientific methods to investigate it, but are capable of undertaking the work required. If there is an obvious gap in your experience give details of others who will be involved with relevant knowledge and experience; some reference to their publications or specialised area of work can be given and again include a copy of a letter from them.

References

Only include those that are central to your proposal, preferably from learned journals. It is important that you have actually read them and have judged their applicability to your project. In the text give the author and the date, e.g. an article by Janet D. Little and Barry R. Seeger in the *Australian Journal of Physiotherapy* would be given as Little and Seeger (1984) in the text, with full details in the reference list. When there are more than two authors it is usual for the name of the first author to be given followed by '*et al.*', e.g. where the four authors of an article in *Physical Therapy* were H. Locke, J. Perry, J. Campbell and L. Thomas, in the text it would be given as Locke *et al.*, (1985).

It is very important to have consistency when writing references. Two systems widely used are the Harvard and Ciba. Examples will illustrate the differences. Choose which suits you but format and punctuation must be similar for all references given. Examples are given first of the Harvard system:

Journal reference
Prior J. A., Webber B. A. (1979). The evaluation of the forced expiration technique as an adjunct to postural drainage. *Physiotherapy*, **65,** (10) 304–307.

Book reference
Kratz C. R. (1978). *Care of the Long Term Sick in the Community*. London: Churchill Livingstone.

The Ciba system has less punctuation.

Journal reference
Duncombe L Howe M C 1985 Group work in occupational therapy: a survey of practice. *American Journal of Occupational Therapy*, **39.3:** 163–170.

2   Applying for funds

There are several sources of research funding open to health professionals; each source has its own method of administration, and in some cases specialist topics may receive priority. The first decision researchers need to make is whether they intend to carry out the research as part of their day-to-day paid employment, if not whether they are seeking money to pay only for equipment and materials or whether all or part of their salary will need to be included. Alternatively, consideration could be given to becoming a student and undertaking research for a higher degree; this can normally be done on a full- or part-time basis.

Personal sources

The clinician who undertakes research while continuing to carry a clinical case load will need to be prepared to work outside normal working hours. It will also be necessary to have the support and interest of the head of the department and other professional colleagues. Being a part-time researcher in a clinical post can be difficult to manage and where a project of any size has been thought through carefully it is sensible to consider applying for full funding. In the conflicting demands for time, clinical work will always have priority over research with the result that the project becomes protracted. The advantage of part-clinical, part-research allocation is that the clinician can get a feel for research without relinquishing contact with patients or clients.

Research post

Posts are advertised in professional journals and often require the researcher in the first instance to learn research skills by working on projects of others. In a research unit where there are a number of different projects under-way there is often a good opportunity to develop ideas. A number of research fellowships are awarded by government agencies and medical organisations in Britain and else-where, but some of these research training opportunities require registration for a research degree at a university or institute of higher education as a prerequisite for awarding the grant.

Health authorities

A number of hospitals and social health foundations have funds which are available to researchers. The situation varies in different countries but funds for health research are usually held by government departments, academic bodies, professional bodies or hospital and specialist centres.

In Britain, regional health authorities have special funds and district hospitals also provide funding for some projects in their own hospital. The Department of Health acts as a grant-awarding body for research funding through a series of research groups. Both the Medical Research Council and the Social Science Research Council support health and social services research, however, they normally require the applicant to have appropriate degrees or previous experience in research before giving funding.

Large organisations publish annual reports of their research activities and these are well worth reading before applying for funding; reports indicate areas of interest in research as well as how systems operate and whom to contact.

A good starting point for any would-be researcher is their own professional body, which should be able to offer advice, and in some instances where research foundations have been set up, direct access to funds.

Charitable bodies

These can form an important source of funding for researchers in the clinical field. Some offer opportunities to train as researchers; advertisements for this are found in the professional journals. Some of the organisations in Britain which have shown particular interest are: The Chest and Heart and Stroke Association, British Rheumatism Association, Spastics Society, Parkinson's Disease Society, National Fund for Research into Crippling Diseases and the Arthritis and Rheumatism Council.

When applying for money it is necessary to consider the approach carefully. Which body is most appropriate for my purpose? What are their interests? Whom can I approach to discuss my ideas informally? What sort of information do they want and which type of application form do they use?

Before sending in your application it is as well to consider the grounds on which it may be judged.

Will you get a grant?
In the opinion of Calnan (1976) referees usually ask themselves five questions about applications for research grants:

1 Is it important?
2 Can it be done?
3 Is the investigator competent to carry out the work?
4 Can it be done in the specified time?
5 Are the costs realistic?

There are a number of reasons why a research grant may be turned down; these include:

1 Poor selection of a research problem, little scientific merit.
2 There will be little interest in the research findings.

3 The aims and objectives or hypotheses of the research are not sound. The field may already have been adequately researched, the variables cannot be measured, or there is ambiguity in the problem statement.
4 Poor or unworkable design and methods.
5 Unrealistic view of the timescale of the research, costs, and personnel involved.

To avoid many of the difficulties described in this chapter it will benefit the researcher to look for a helpful research adviser and to visit and talk to people in the funding agencies before submitting proposals. A researcher is expected to be a politician in addition to therapist, clinician, manager, specialist and educator!

Reference

Calnan J. (1976). *One Way to Do Research*. London: William Heinemann Medical Books.

6 Organisation of Research

Successful research is dependent on good organisational skills. Many clinicians have basic experience of these skills from running a case load, and helping with departmental management; but it must be remembered that time scales in research are much longer than those in clinical practice.

Organisation involves planning a comprehensive timetable. Some examples are given below but the time taken at each stage will depend on the experience of the researcher, the facilities available, and how much time is available each week for the research.

The reader who has never carried out research will usually underestimate both the time and the resources needed, particularly cost, and this can cause havoc. There are a number of pitfalls to watch out for while organising research.

Time

Research usually takes longer to carry out than is anticipated at the start. Taking the literature search as an example, it is necessary to visit a number of libraries and get to know the librarians. Books and journals may have to be ordered and can take several days or weeks to arrive. The literature then has to be read and relevant information extracted before writing a review. Six months might easily be required for this stage.

Time planning is often subject to factors outside the researcher's control. Funding and ethical committees may only meet two or three times a year, and the experts you want to consult may be on a lecture tour of the USA, Australia or Britain at the time you want to contact them. Special equipment which needs building or modifying to fit the purpose of the research can take a long time to supply.

The sample for one study was to be 100 stroke patients followed up over six months after discharge from hospital. The researchers did not anticipate that it could take at least one year or more to get the 100 patients referred to them and that the six-month follow-up would continue until six months after the last patient entered the sample. The original proposal for six months' preparation, six months for data collection, and six months for analysis and writing up soon became four years!

Costs

While some health and social service institutions are supportive of research, and may be willing to lose the hidden costs of staff carrying out projects, others are not. It is a healthy exercise, even for researchers who will not need to find a funding agency, to calculate the costs of the research. For those who will need funding this is essential. Costs can be difficult to estimate and are generally more than you think they will be at the start. A short questionnaire administered to 50 patients can involve paying postal costs, secretarial services and photocopying. The cost of travelling to see patients at home or even to visit libraries soon mounts up. Multiple copies of final reports are important as research findings should be disseminated as widely as possible, but this leads to additional costs. Inadequate costing and incorrect financial claims can seriously endanger the completion of the project. Remember that you will not be given the sum you apply for at the start of the project. The amount you estimate for will be available to be claimed as needed from the grant-holding institution.

Cooperation

A beautifully designed and written research proposal is useless unless professional staff, patients, clients and their relatives are willing to cooperate with the researcher in carrying out the practical work. When setting up the fieldwork, time must be spent in informing *all* the people who may be affected by the research about its purpose and allowing them to comment on any procedures which may involve them. The following example illustrates this.

> In a study of dressing ability carried out with a group of hospitalised rheumatoid patients, the nursing staff were not informed of the nature of the research and the importance of their cooperation. This led to the situation where nursing staff did not have patients washed, breakfasted and ready for dressing practice at 09.00. One objective of the research was to test morning dressing capacity.

In addition to informing patients and other professional groups, it is often equally important to explain the purpose of the research to other health service personnel such as porters, ambulancemen, and domestic staff. On occasion it may be necessary to notify union representatives about your research if it is seen to have implications for peoples' jobs. Hospital administrators should be informed about any research being undertaken. Try to send out letters at the same time, as negative feelings about the project can be aroused if someone who will be involved feels they 'haven't been told' and other people inform them about the proposed study. A more extensive discussion of clinical considerations in research is given in Chapter 7.

Availability of subjects

Research cannot be carried out without subjects, yet at any gathering of clinical researchers there will be a sad tale of the 'disappearing' client. Many studies have been set up where the clinician has encountered problems in finding enough subjects to complete the research regardless of whether this is stroke patients, patients with a Colles' fracture, bilateral amputees, or people with anorexia nervosa. It would appear that because patients in some of these diagnostic categories take up so much treatment time in a department, it is believed that there are many of them around to take part in the research.

Records need careful checking to establish just how many stroke or other group of patients have been admitted to a hospital over the previous 12 months, and of these how many were atypical and could not be included in a sample.

Elderly people can present particular difficulty for the researcher who has to consider how many may die or become too ill to cooperate during the period of the research. One therapist was interested in looking at factors leading to falls in an elderly population in a residential home. She wanted to investigate 25 residents but realising there might be a considerable dropout rate aimed to get 35 patients into the study. In the end she was able to monitor 23 residents over a ten-month period.

How many subjects do I need in my study?
This is a question that everyone wants to know and the frequent answer given 'how long is a piece of string?' is infuriating. However, there is no easy answer, and frequently you have to make do with the number available, the problem is nearly always finding a sufficient number. If you are investigating in a new area, studying either patient or client groups, or treatment and management techniques, a good starting point may be a single case study design (*see* Chapter 4). You can then familiarise yourself with different aspects of the problem before starting on a larger study.

The number of subjects you can obtain will of course depend on those available. A look at records may give you some idea of how many of the particular group you want were available over the past year or six months. But records are often poorly kept and the estimate obtained from them may not be very accurate and may overestimate the number that will actually be available.

If you are studying a problem that occurs fairly rarely you cannot expect many subjects. For example conditions such as arthrogryposis or motor neurone disease are not nearly so commonly found as arthropathies or patients with psychiatric problems.

Probably having less than 20 patients/clients overall will mean that you are really only undertaking a pilot study as a preliminary to something larger. One of the problems is that if you start off with 20 subjects and divide into two groups for comparison you are immediately down to ten in each group. If you want to divide them further, for example on the basis of age, sex or seriousness of condition, you are down to five in each group.

One way to have more subjects in your group is to undertake a multicentre study, but this will increase many other problems. It is necessary to monitor that everyone is doing exactly the same thing, and the general organisation of such a project may extend the length of the study by years. This should really only be tackled by an experienced researcher.

Another way to increase the number of subjects is for several people to agree to undertake similar studies each in their area. Thus three people each collecting 20 subjects can give a respectable total of 60.

There is a statistical formula for finding out how many patients you need in an experimental study if you want your results to be able to show a statistical difference, if one exists. Consultation with a statistician is essential at this stage, but before you meet do think about the kind of change you expect in your subjects, and the degree of change you would consider it was, in real life terms, important to detect. For example in examining degrees of range of movement, you may consider that changes of two or three degrees really have no practical meaning, but you want to detect any change above, say, ten degrees.

People often start to say very early on in a study 'how many people do I need?' But this is a question which comes later, after you have established your objectives, hypotheses and the research design. The research design you select will help to decide the appropriate number of subjects to include.

Supervision of research work

If someone agrees to supervise the research project or help with particular aspects of the work, it is advisable to agree and actually spell out exactly what that supervision or help will involve. An academic may agree to supervise, and presume this means looking at the research proposal, having an occasional chat and looking at the results before they are written up. 'Supervision' to the researcher may have meant hourly visits every week. It saves later embarrassment and disappointment to discuss exactly what supervision or help is going to mean at an early stage.

Organisation of data

An information and filing system should be set up at the same time that the research idea starts to be explored. All references, correspondence, and telephone messages should be systematically recorded. Failure to do this can lead to frustration and chaos. A daily diary can also be helpful. This part of the organisation is in addition to handling data collection and analysis. Failure to adopt a comprehensive filing system can lead to the following frustrations.

Having to repeat the literature search because some of the details needed for the final report are missing, such as year of publication of some articles.

Having to read lengthy articles or books again to find out where important sentences or examples are, which were the basis of the research aims and objectives.

Not being able to follow up some of the people in the sample because their change of address was written on the back of an envelope which was later thrown away.

Before the data you have collected can be analysed they have to be organised into a manageable form. Different procedures may be appropriate. A summary table (Table 6.1) can provide a useful way of organising the information as a first step; for example, for different questions give totals to each answer.

Table 6.1   Summary Tables

Question 1 Have you ever had a stroke before?	Yes	No	DK	NA
	89	39	12	60

Question 10 How often does the district nurse visit?	Frequently	Occasionally	Not at all	NA
	51	80	29	40

Total no. of subjects = 200

DK = Do not know. NA = Not applicable. These two need to be distinguished from each other and from a straight 'no' answer.

Coding frame

If you have a large amount of data or if you propose to use a computer for analysing the data a coding frame must be constructed. This means that all possible responses to each question must be assigned a number. The numbers do not have real meaning but enable you to identify each response to each question. This, like so many research tasks, is not complicated but needs to be carried out meticulously, making sure every possible answer is categorised. It is always important to differentiate between no, do not know (DK) and not applicable (NA) as they can imply very different things. Before making out the coding frame you need to study some of your forms and find the kind of answers that have been given and what they mean.

Where you have open questions these may be dealt with by content analysis (for details *see* Chapter 10), or you may be able to classify the answers into a number of categories with perhaps a small 'other' category. The examples given below are taken from a survey of physiotherapy in the community.

Question 12 *Place of treatment* Week 1	1 = Patient's own home 2 = GP premises 3 = Health centre 4 = Residential home 5 = School 6 = Combination 7 = Other
Question 13 *Main reason for place of treatment*	0 = No main reason 1 = Patient medically unfit 2 = Difficult to get patient out 3 = Treatment related to home 4 = Long distance to hospital 5 = Long delay in hospital 6 = Nearest place 7 = Other 9 = NA

A full coding frame needs to be drawn up which lists everything from the subject's name or number, each question or measurement to be used, and each possible response to the question or measurement, each specified by number. It is helpful to look at other researchers' coding frames to see how a completed one looks. Your draft coding frame can act as a basis for discussion with the statistician.

In this chapter, a number of diverse aspects of research organisation have been discussed ranging from the costs of research and sample selection to the procedures for grouping data. All the topics have in common the need for good management skills; clinicians should not feel daunted by this as many of the skills of research have already been developed in the clinical field.

7 Ethics

Ethical matters are particularly important in research and often involve difficult decisions. Most research raises some ethical issues and considering them at an early stage helps to avoid problems later on. It is not always clear what is meant by the term ethics, but the definition given in the *Concise Oxford English Dictionary* (1984) covers most aspects: 'relating to morals, treating moral questions, morally correct, honourable'. Many countries have medical bodies concerned with ethics in research, the American Medical Association and the Medical Research Councils of Britain and Canada issue guidelines (American Medical Association, 1966; Medical Research Council, 1963; Medical Research Council, 1966).

In this chapter there is discussion of ethical issues that arise in different stituations where research is being undertaken; functions of ethical committees whose permission must usually be obtained before starting a project are also described.

Clinicians undertaking research

The main ethical issue for clinicians is the safeguarding of patients' interests. It is essential that before anyone is included in any research project as a subject he or she must have given free and informed consent to take part. A good definition of what this means is given by the British Medical Research Council (1963) in their Guidelines on Ethics:

> Consent freely given with proper understanding of the nature and consequences of what is proposed. Assumed consent or consent obtained by undue influences is valueless and in this latter respect particular care is necessary when the volunteer stands in special relationships to the investigator, as in the case of a patient to his doctor.

It is as well to check that information on the following points has been given so that consent can be informed.

1 The purpose of the study.
2 The identity of the research worker and the organisation funding the study if there is one.
3 How he or she as an individual was selected for the study.
4 The measures that have been taken to safeguard the confidentiality of information given, and the assurance that no identification of any individual will be possible when the study is reported.
5 Exactly what 'full participation' means, i.e. the proposed duration of the study and where appropriate the frequency and length of individual sessions.
6 What involvement in the study will actually entail, e.g. observation during treatment sessions, physical examination, the type of treatments that will be given and, where appropriate, the methods of allocation to different treatment groups should be explained.

It can often be difficult for a patient to refuse to participate in anything proposed by those responsible for their care and treatment. Requests should be worded so that refusal is not difficult for the patient and does not cause them unnecessary apprehension. Acquiescence must never be taken for granted.

Finally it must be emphasised to the patient that he has the absolute right to opt out at any time, for any or no reason.

It is wise to obtain consent in a formal manner and if there is a possibility of misunderstanding it is advisable to obtain written consent, but remember that this in itself can be unsettling for some elderly patients; signing forms can have worrying implications. The overriding concern should be to avoid any unnecessary stress to patients or their relatives.

If, for some reason, the patient is unable to understand the implications of participation, then informed consent should be obtained from relatives or legal guardians. Greater sensitivity may be needed for patients with problems of communication and comprehension, ensuring that they are not distressed by any procedures.

Permission from the medical practitioners responsible for the care of patients who might be included in the study must be obtained at an early stage before the study commences; they will need to have full information about the purpose and proposed methods. There is no obligation for any doctor to agree, and his final decision must be respected. It is also as well to find out if the patient is currently involved in any other study as if so there might be a conflict of interests.

All others concerned with the care of the patients in the study, such as nurses, or other therapists, should be contacted individually at an early stage, hospital administrators should also be informed. Efforts should be made by the research worker at the planning stage to ensure that hospital and departmental routines are disturbed as little as possible. It is important to try to obtain the enthusiastic cooperation of all those whose work might be affected by the study, by convincing them of the value of the work you are undertaking.

Patient records

Some research may involve the examination or analysis of existing records rather than involving patients themselves. Permission to extract and use information must be obtained from the doctor or other clinician who made the records and from the medical records department. An undertaking should be given in writing to the head of the medical records department, naming individuals who will have access to the records and describing the procedures that have been devised to ensure there will be no disclosure of confidential information in written or verbal form.

Physical security of the information must be ensured by using locked cabinets; identifying data such as names or addresses should be kept separately from the main body of the records. A system of numbers or codes can be used to identify individual records.

Any confidential material should be destroyed by shredding or burning when no longer needed. Confidentiality is

an overriding principle in investigations with human subjects. Lack of attention to these matters is not only unethical but will also damage your reputation as a researcher.

The use of healthy volunteers

Studies are often undertaken to examine aspects of 'normal'
populations. The principles in the last two sections apply
equally here: informed consent must be obtained and
participants assured of the confidential procedures that will
be applied to information obtained. If there is any possibility that potentially dangerous procedures will be used, not
only must the risks be clearly stated but written consent
obtained.

Other considerations

There are a number of other issues which should be
clarified at an early stage to avoid later problems. When
collaborating with others the apportioning of the work
must be clearly agreed and it is wise to discuss who the
major author of the final report will be. The author whose
name appears first is assumed to be the researcher who has
undertaken the major role, not the person of most senior
rank. If there are several researchers who have made a
major contribution to the work or the report, the conven-
tion is for their names to be given alphabetically—it is hard
lines if your name is Zacharia!

When writing the research report it is important to
present the findings clearly and honestly, not only avoiding
false statements but also revealing facts which may not
support the research hypotheses; clear separation of fact
from opinion is not only responsible but sensible, as there
will be less grounds for criticism if you yourself identify not
only the strengths but also the weaknesses of the study. It
could be argued that it is unethical to be involved in badly
planned, poorly designed research, as it is unlikely to
produce any useful results, and both time and money will
have been misused.

Assisting in research

Clinicians practising in hospitals, departments and clinics where research is being undertaken by others may find themselves becoming involved in ethical issues. They may be asked to take part in a number of different ways, by being observed at work, assisting in data collection, or delivering treatments or procedures that are part of a project. Anyone involved in any of those ways must be confident that the procedures necessary to safeguard the patient's interests, which have been discussed earlier in this chapter, have been put into action. It is also worth considering if anything in the protocol contravenes professional ethics. This situation can be a delicate one for the clinician, with conflict between clinical and research interests; if participation is clearly having an adverse effect on the patient, the clinician's overriding commitment is to the patient's welfare. It may be necessary to represent the patient's wishes to the researcher, possibly enlisting support from other senior clinicians. Patients may more readily confide their fears about the effects of the research to the person treating them.

The clinician who is asked to assist in data collection has a dual role to consider. Professional ethics state that there is a first principle, 'all information acquired in the course of work should be held in confidence'. Confidentiality of information is essential; information available through clinical work cannot be made available to the research team unless previously agreed with the patient and others concerned with the patient's care; similarly any data collected for research purposes cannot be made available to other clinicians. With careful planning and forethought these problems can be resolved.

Superintendents and managers of services

Those involved in organising services may find themselves in a position where staff in their own department are involved or wish to become involved in research, or others outside their area wish to use patients or staff as subjects of their investigation. In either case the persons responsible for the service must concern themselves with several ethical issues about the patients, the staff and the running of the department or clinic.

It is the responsibility of those undertaking the research to provide evidence to the manager that ethical issues have been given due consideration in the planning of the study; that informed consent will be obtained and the patients' rights carefully safeguarded. A copy of the written protocol which outlines these matters should be available. The exact extent of the involvement of clinical staff must be known before approval for the work to start is given. It is dangerous to agree to participate without seeing a written protocol—if this is not forthcoming it is wise for the manager to write to the researchers restating any verbal agreement and describing exactly the conditions under which participation has been agreed.

The rights of staff must be protected too; if there is a heavy clinical load the extra work of an outside project may place too much strain on individual clinicians and their health, and the care of patients, may suffer.

Research undertaken in a department or clinic will reflect on that department, so if poor research work is allowed to proceed, it will only bring disrepute on all those concerned.

Ethical committees

Most hospitals and clinics have committees which look into ethical matters related to investigations involving human subjects, and act as a review body. One of their tasks is to examine research protocols to see if the procedures proposed safeguard such matters as patient safety, patient rights, and confidentiality of information. Without permission from these committees projects cannot go ahead. It is worthwhile taking time in your application to the committee to spell out clearly ways in which you have ensured that ethical issues have been given due attention. Remember that these committees often meet infrequently, possibly only every three or six months. Personal contact with a member of the committee, to obtain guidance on the specific information that the committee requires, may be useful.

Check that jargon is omitted from the proposal as members of the committee may come from a wide range of professions and also include people from outside the health care field.

References

American Medical Association (1966) *Ethical Guidelines for Clinical Investigations*. Chicago: Chicago American Medical Association.

Medical Research Council (1963) *Responsibility in Investigations on Human Subjects*. Reprinted from the Report of the Medical Research Council 1962/3 (Cmnd 2382) pp. 21–25.

Medical Research Council (1966) *Extra-Mural Programmes*. Ottawa, Canada: Medical Research Council.

8 Methods of Data Collection

When asked about their proposed study the inexperienced researcher may say 'I am going to send out a questionnaire', or 'I am going to measure range of movement of the shoulder'. The reader of this book will see that it has taken seven chapters of careful preparation before the selection of the data collection method can be made. The aims, objectives and research design will all help to indicate how the data should be collected.

In Chapter 5 several research designs were discussed and examples given of five different types of study: retrospective, descriptive, clinical, experimental and single case study design. While in some cases the selection of the design indicates the precise method of data collection to be used, in others it does not. An example of the latter is when selecting a descriptive design in which observational methods may be adopted. Here in addition to observation, data from interviews, questionnaires, and measurements of particular functions may also be needed.

1 Using written information from existing records and reports

Before setting up a system to collect new data, the clinician should consider using data which are already available in clinical records and reports. Much of this will have been gathered for administrative or treatment purposes, and will range from accurate to highly unreliable information. The researcher will have a fair idea of the accuracy of the information that has been collected in their own department, but cross-checking will be necessary where the status of the records is unknown. It is not unusual to find a patient's age or even diagnosis changing across the records from one department to another. There is often a descending order of reliability depending on the use to which the records are put. Hence ambulance services may be good for addresses, outpatient records for age and date of admission, ward notes for diagnosis and medication, and therapy records for physical progress and functional ability. Even here you may find much data missing.

The researcher may need to set up recording systems which are specifically designed for the research. Where this is the case, it is necessary to train, encourage, and supervise the people who help to complete them. The design and instructions which go with record-keeping forms are very important. They should always be kept simple and unambiguous as in the following example.

Please enter the patient's details on their first attendance.

Patient's name:
  Mr/Mrs/Miss   Surname .... Forenames ....

Date of birth:

Date of first attendance:

Main diagnosis for which patient referred for treatment (from patient's medical notes)

....

---

2   Observation

In making assessments and planning treatment programmes clinicians rely heavily on watching their patients' behaviour. They are skilled observers, and these skills can be used in research. However, for research purposes objective ways of recording observations need to be found so that bias can be controlled. This can be done by using independent observers, or by recording the behaviour on tape recorders or film so that it can be checked by other people at a later date. Data collection through observation can be either participant observation, where the researcher joins in the action and then records events later, or non-participant observation, where the researcher stands aside to observe the action and records it as it happens.

Both these approaches can provide rich data, but skill and tact are needed to operate them successfully as can be seen in the following examples.

Example   *Participant observation*

A study was carried out of group activities in one ward of a large psychiatric hospital. The patient group was told that the psychologist was carrying out a study of non-verbal behaviour in groups and would be recording what had happened after each session. The participants were reassured that they would be able to see and comment on any data collected. Despite this 'honest' approach, the patients and staff in the group reported that they felt 'watched' and that they found it difficult to behave normally. They were much happier when the researcher was replaced by a video camera.

Example   *Non-participant observation*

The study was carried out in a residential home for physically disabled adults. The researcher wanted to keep an accurate time log of when certain activities took place: feeding, toiletting, bathing, and movement between rooms. The residents agreed to take part in the study, and knew that someone would be discreetly wandering round the home filling in boxes on a sheet of paper attached to a clipboard. The residents found that the novelty of being watched wore off after the first day, and the staff, despite reassurance to the contrary, worried that a time and motion study was being carried out of their work.

In therapy departments observation is common behaviour and as such is seen as legitimate by most patients. Even so, patients must be told when they are being used as subjects for research despite any difference in behaviour which may result. Practice 'dry' runs where the subjects get used to being observed are often a help.

3   Interviews

Interviewing is widely used in research to gather information and to assess subjects' physical, social, emotional and intellectual functions. An interview is a 'conversation with a purpose', but the directness with which this purpose is pursued varies according to the interviewer's primary goal and the objectives of the study.

The amount of structure in an interview varies from a totally unstructured interview with probe questions, which can be useful in the early stages of research, through to a fully structured interview where the same questions are asked in the same order using the same wording for each interviewee. Both types of interviews are used by researchers for data collection. People will often give extensive information in an informal interview that they would be reluctant to have tape recorded or to write down, but the method can lead to difficulty in handling and analysing the quantity of interview material. The skilled interviewer has to learn to run the interview without personal involvement and clinicians have to learn to use rather a different technique from that used for interviewing as part of assessment for treatment. The interview technique has limitations. The influence of the interviewer may affect the answers given and distortion of facts can result from the interpretations of the interviewer. A number of interview biases have been identified and these are well documented in interviewers' handbooks and research method books. They include the following:

Social desirability

The individual desires respect and may wish to please and be accepted by the interviewer. He may distort facts to achieve these ends, either consciously or unconsciously.

Conforming

The individual may think that he should conform to the attitudes and values of the interviewer. 'I think that all the staff in the hospitals are underpaid for the wonderful work they do.'

Stereotyping

The interviewer may form a faulty impression of the interviewee because of his clothes, accent or mannerisms.

'Halo' effect

The interviewer may allow his perception of one characteristic of the interviewee, usually positive, to influence his interpretation of other aspects, the first impression often having the strongest effect.

All these factors can affect the reliability of interviews, but being aware of them can help to compensate for these biases.

Despite the evidence for the unreliability of interviews there are many good reasons for its continued use. Among these is the fact that it allows many sorts of information to be collected which would be difficult to collect in any other way. Interviews also have an exploratory function: for example, gathering information about which the interviewer need not have preconceived ideas. Also, as this is an exchange situation, information can be given as well as received.

There are several guides to interview techniques available which provide constructive guidelines to reliable interview practices, and some books are suggested in the Bibliography.

4 Projective techniques

Where data collection is by observation or interview, the subjects reveal their behaviour directly to the researcher. Some people are unwilling or unable to do this in such a concrete way, and researchers may find that projective techniques are appropriate, particularly in psychiatry or with young children. Creative writing, art, play, and music can be used in addition to the better known projective tests such as the Rorschach test, the Minnesota Multiphasic Personality Inventory (MMPI), and the Goodenough Draw-a-man test. These latter tests can only be used by people who are trained and skilled in their use, usually a psychologist. If you as a clinician want to use these kinds of techniques, a psychologist may have to be included in the research team.

Projective techniques are designed to look at personality structure and the adaptive responses of an individual. They may be used to indicate change in response to treatment over time. However, the researcher must be very cautious when using projective techniques because they include a high subjective element. They should only be used in conjunction with other more objective methods of investigation.

5 Questionnaires and schedules

Questionnaires are not in themselves a method of data collection, they are the instrument with which data are collected. They may be used as part of interviews and projective techniques, but are most commonly used for carrying out surveys. The information gained through surveys can be used in a variety of ways by a number of people. It may be an administrator who wants to know about the use of a casualty department, the number of patients attending, the type of problems they present with, and the number of staff on duty at different times of the day. It may be a therapist who wants to investigate attitudes of students towards elderly patients or a nurse interested in career patterns of nurses after obtaining state registration.

The term questionnaire is usually used to describe self-completion sheets, while schedules refers to those completed in face-to-face interviews. Schedules completed at interview can either be structured, all the question wordings are uniform and standardised and the responses often precoded; or open, where the subject matter is specified but the interviewer asks a question to which there can be an extensive range of responses. In practice, many interview schedules combine the two approaches, in this case the researcher needs to remember that the data collected from open-ended questions are harder to handle and analyse than those from structured questions. A rule of thumb is that open-ended questions are most useful at the exploratory stage of a study, or where feelings, attitudes and motives are involved. Structured questions are more appropriate when obtaining factual information from a large-scale population.

These examples of closed and open questions are taken from a study of physiotherapy services in the community.

Closed questions
Do you have easy access to the patient's clinical notes?   No ☐
                                                           Yes ☐
Sex: male   ☐
      female   ☐
Marital status: single   ☐
                 married   ☐
                 other   ☐
If you have children, please indicate numbers in the following age groups:
0–4 years   ☐
5–15 years   ☐
16 years and over   ☐

Open questions
Can you suggest any other aspects of your physiotherapy service outside hospital that might be improved? ....

What specific benefit to patients is provided by your physiotherapy service outside hospital? ....

Please make any further comments, if you wish, on the advantages or disadvantages of your present physiotherapy service, both for the patients and for you as a physiotherapist ....

Use simple language   Does the patient understand terms such as cerebrovascular accident or menisectomy?

Use simple questions   Keep them as short as possible and introduce one theme at a time. Does the patient understand the question: 'In the event of your wife dying and no hospital bed being available for several weeks, would you prefer to be looked after solely by staff from the Good Neighbours scheme or a combination of the District Nurse and the Home Help?'

Avoid the following:

Ambiguity   'Is your housework made more difficult because you have had a stroke?'

'No' answers to this could be: No, housework is not more difficult because my family won't let me do it/I don't do it any more/The Home Help does it/I don't have any difficulty.

Vague words   'Since having your stroke are you still able to get out regularly?'

There is no indication of what is meant by regularly. Regularly for one person could be the monthly visit to her daughter who lives some distance away, for another the daily visit to the corner shop.

Leading questions   'Do you agree that community physiotherapy is important?'

This wording will bias the answers towards positive responses.

'Do you have any aids such as a bath seat or walking frame?'

People who are unsure about their responses to this will tend to seek refuge in the suggestions given; to overcome this either all or none of the alternatives should be stated.

Presuming questions   Questions that imply that the respondent has knowledge or an opinion about a topic.

'What is your opinion about hospital versus community care?'

Hypothetical questions   'Would you like to live in a flat?'

Most people say they are willing to try anything once, but an affirmative answer to this question would be unlikely to predict future behaviour.

Personal or embarrassing questions   These can be related to money, age, sex or other items of significance to the person being interviewed. Some topics may be too personal for an individual to discuss. If the topic is a potentially sensitive one extra care must be given to wording and layout of questions.

Questions involving memory   'How often have you visited your doctor during the last year?' It is doubtful whether many people could answer this question accurately.

The space provided may limit the length of responses to open questions or you may wish to provide additional sheets of blank paper.

When designing questions for questionnaires and schedules, the type of question, the wording and instructions for the interviewer must all be considered carefully and very explicit instructions given. Pitfalls are often readily identified once the schedule is in use and that is why pilot work is essential. Some of the most important points to consider are given on p. 67.

When designing a questionnaire or schedule it is essential to have the information you want listed out in detail before you start thinking of the questions you will actually ask. This is necessary so that when you are designing the question wording you can check back to your information list to find whether the responses to the questions will give you the data you want.

Whichever form of data collection is adopted, the researcher must set up an organised system for recording and storing information. Otherwise it is possible to reach a stage in your research when desks, tables and floors can be covered with unidentifiable paperwork.

9 Tools of Measurement

When the research question has been clearly defined and the research design selected, consideration will have to be given to the tools of measurement that will be needed. Clinicians often use their subjective judgement when assessing and measuring aspects of their patient's performance, but for a research project any methods of measurement used must be demonstrably free from subjective bias, and be both valid and reliable. (These two terms are described fully in the Glossary.) Briefly, to be valid a test must be shown to measure what it purports to measure, and to be reliable it must be shown to give consistent results when used by different people, and by the same person on different occasions.

In professions that lack a long-standing tradition of research, valid and reliable methods of measurement are not readily available, and one of the reasons why clinical research is often criticised, and rightly so, is because not enough attention has been given in the past to selecting appropriate tools of measurement. The whole value of your work can be jeopardised if insufficient attention is given to this aspect.

First it is important to search the literature and find what tools of measurement are available in the area in which you are interested. Examine those you find carefully and see what evidence is given for their reliability and validity when used with different groups. If a standardised test is available remember that the validity and reliability of the test only apply if you follow procedures given in the accompanying manuals. If you decide to use only some of the questions or alter it in some way you will need to retest it yourself to find if it is still reliable in the adapted format.

Even if you are using a straightforward method of measurement, for example a hand-held goniometer, it is still important to find out the range of error when it is used by different people and to specify clearly conditions under which measurement is going to take place, for example 'with the subject fully supported lying prone having rested for five minutes prior to measurement'. Specifying time of day may also be important where repeated measurements are carried out.

Discuss your needs with other researchers who may know of suitable tools of measurement. If you really cannot find anything suitable for your purpose you will have to consider developing a tool specifically for your study. This is extremely time consuming and you will certainly need help from others with particular expertise in this area.

A researcher at the British Department of Health was looking for a measure of disability and soon came across activities of daily living scales (ADLS) commonly used in occupational therapy departments. In a matter of weeks he uncovered over 200 variations in use around the country, few had any instructions about how to fill them in, and there was little evidence of their reliability when used by different people or the same person on different occasions. There was also little evidence that they were used repeatedly to monitor change but rather on a one-off basis and then filed away. Despite this 'dustbin' approach there have been a number of attempts to produce a standardised ADL scale.

The clinician who finds that he must develop his own measuring instrument will need to adopt the following procedure:

1 Select the function, behaviour, or service to be measured.
2 Define all terms used fully and unambiguously. For example mobility or disability need clear and explicit definitions for the purpose of the study.
3 Look at other tools available, describe their characteristics and the type of items used.
4 Design a prototype instrument.
5 Pilot the prototype instrument on a sample population, ask others to do the same for you.
6 Carry out statistical and other tests on the results to

ensure that it is both valid and reliable. An example of this preliminary kind of work is given by Mathiowetz *et al.* (1985).

The main point here is that reliability or validity must never be assumed. Even well known scales frequently used, such as the Barthel Index (Mahoney and Barthel, 1965) and that devised by Fugl-Meyer *et al.* (1975) do not, in these published versions, give evidence that items are mutually exclusive 1–4 that is, that all observers or researchers using the scale with the same patients will all independently give each subject the same score. Reliable scoring of the scale is essential.

Therapists are familiar with performance categories such as: independent; needs verbal help; needs help of one person; needs help of two people; and, cannot do, and often feel that they adequately reflect levels of independence of their elderly or disabled patients. But does this really reflect individual performance? Does it matter who gives the help? One can often see an experienced therapist giving minimal help to a patient transferring from bed to chair, but it may require two or even three inexperienced helpers. And 'cannot do', because a patient does not perform an activity when requested could reflect not only 'ability' but the extent of the patient's motivation to comply with instructions. If he does not do it on one occasion it must not be assumed that he 'cannot'. Another assumption that is often made is that if numbers are assigned to levels of performance these numbers have numerical values and can be added together to give a meaningful total, for example:

Independent	3
Needs a little help	2
Needs a lot of help	1
Does not do	0

But these numbers do not have real meaning in the sense that the intervals between them have meaning. They are an example of a nominal scale (*see* Glossary). As it stands the numbers mean no more than those on an athlete's vest! A method of measurement useful in research which therapists often find particularly difficult is the YES/NO answer.

Does the patient stand independently?	YES	NO
Does the patient walk six steps without the help of another person?	YES	NO

Because therapy is usually concerned with quality of performance this crude measurement seems inadequate but in the end, in real life terms, what everyone needs to know is 'is the patient able to perform the activity safely on his/her own?'

In summary, valid and reliable forms of measurement are an essential part of any experimental investigation, and testing and developing them may be a necessary first stage in many projects. It may also form the basis for a complete project.

References

Fugl-Meyer A. R., Jääsicö L., Leyman I., Olsson S., Steglind S. (1975). The post-stroke hemiplegic patient. *Scandinavian Journal of Rehabilitation Medicine*, **7**, 13–31.

Mahoney F. I., Barthel D. W. (1965). Functional evaluation: the Barthel Index. *Maryland State Medical Journal*, Feb, 61–65.

Mathiowetz V., Volland G., Kashman N., Weber K. (1985). Adult norms for the box and block test of manual dexterity. *American Journal of Occupational Therapy*, **39**, 386–391.

10 Analysis and Presentation of Results

For some people statistics seem to be of central importance in their research and they devote much time and energy to 'playing' with their data, but while an understanding of statistical analysis is essential for some investigations, for many small clinical studies little statistical analysis is needed in presenting the results. Clear data presentation will be the critical feature.

The purpose of statistical analysis was originally to present information on large sets of data in a comprehensive way, and to test assumptions about relationships between different sets of data. In clinical studies such relationships could be the date of onset of a disease and time of admission to hospital for treatment, or the scores obtained of some measure of functional ability before and after treatment.

In studies where small numbers of subjects are used, and aims and objectives 'specified' rather than 'hypothesised', the results can often be presented clearly by use of graphs, pie charts and histograms, using raw data. The readers are then able to assess for themselves the soundness of the conclusions the researcher draws from the data. Examples are given of some of these ways of presenting data—graph (Fig. 10.1), pie chart (Fig. 10.2), histogram (Fig. 10.3) and tables (Tables 10.1 and 10.2). Note that headings, number of subjects and identification of the axes should always be given.

Although these simple methods of presenting data are often appropriate it may sometimes be necessary to consider other forms of data analysis, particularly when collecting a large amount of information. The most important question when considering statistical analysis is to decide

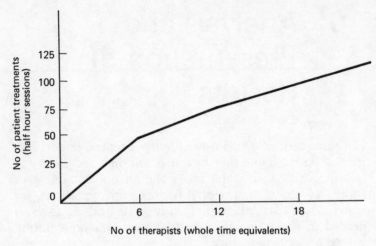

Fig. 10.1   *Graph—to show the relationship between the number of therapists in post and the number of patient treatments per week.*

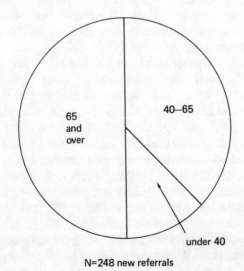

Fig. 10.2   *Pie chart—showing the ages of patients referred to a therapy department during one calendar year.*

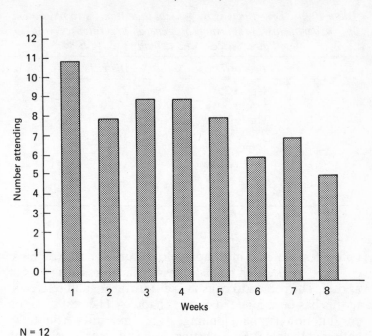

N = 12

Fig. 10.3   *Histogram—showing the number of patients attending a weekly relaxation class over an eight-week period.*

Table 10.1.   *Physiotherapists' reasons given for taking up present post*

Reasons	Main	Secondary	Additional
Wanted to work in the community	17	5	
Hours suited family commitments	10	12	
Able to work near home	9	1	4
Able to work without supervision		6	5
Other	2	6	6
Total	38		
n = 38.			

Table 10.2. Direct access by general practitioners to physiotherapy departments: proportion of general practitioners who are offered direct access who actually use it (1984)

Proportions	Districts
Up to 25%	9
Up to 50%	20
Up to 75%	30
75–95%	23
100%	58
Don't know	12
	152

on the test which is most appropriate for the data you have collected, and which helps to answer the questions you are asking. The person to consult is a statistician, and reference to this has been made in earlier chapters. The best time for consultation is the planning stage—not after you have collected the data! The questions you will want to ask about your data are usually concerned with similarities and differences. For example, can I assume that these two groups of patients randomly selected are similar? To what extent do the disability scores obtained on a test in a hospital or clinic correlate with disability in the home? Are the scores obtained by a treated and untreated group of patients significantly different?

It is important to seek help at an early stage because the analysis you want to perform on the data will decide the way in which it has to be collected. But do remember to have absolutely clear in your own mind what you want from your data before you consult a statistician, otherwise you may fall into the trap of undertaking complex analyses which may be statistically possible but nonsense in real life terms in relation to your data. It is also important to distinguish 'real life' significance from 'statistical' significance—they may be very different, as the following example shows.

In a study of the efficacy of chest physiotherapy and intermittent positive pressure breathing in the resolution of pneumonia by Graham and Bradley (1978), the conclusion was that chest physiotherapy and intermittent positive pressure breathing do not hasten resolution of pneumonia. However, most therapists would not consider physiotherapy had a place in the treatment of acute pneumonia. The lack of statistically significant differences between treated and untreated groups was not of real life 'significance' or importance.

This book does not attempt to explain statistical analysis, the reader is referred to a number of suitable texts in the Bibliography, but a superficial description of the tests most commonly used in clinical studies may be helpful to those reading research papers. Three groups of tests are briefly described.

1 Those that try to find if the differences observed between two sets of scores are significantly different, i.e. what is the probability that these differences are due to the research procedure or could they have been obtained by chance?

The student t-test and chi square (or χ^2) are tests which are used in a 'before and after' test situation. For example, are the scores on some test taken before and after treatment significantly different? They might also be used when you want to know whether two groups of patients were similar or not. For example, when examining the effect of ADL dressing sessions on the populations of two geriatric wards, you might want to examine in advance, by the use of a test, whether or not the populations in the two wards were significantly different or whether you could assume they were similar for the purposes of the trial. The starting point for the study, if you were going to give one ward the benefit of a special therapy intervention, would be to ensure that the overall levels of independent dressing were similar in the two wards, though patients themselves might appear to differ.

2 Those that examine two sets of scores to find the extent of correlation between them. The two sets of scores might be scores from one set of individuals, or from two different groups. Your interest is in finding if one score goes up or down, whether the corresponding one also does. You want to find out how closely the scores covary, and whether in a positive or negative way. You might want to know if depression was related to performance of functional activities. In that case you could use a correlation test to examine the relationship between scores on a word adjective checklist and a performance test— remembering, of course, that any relationship demonstrated through the use of these tests is *correlational* and not *causal*. In the example above, if a positive correlation is demonstrated between word scores and performance test scores it does not necessarily mean that poor performance is caused by depression (*see* Glossary for discussion on correlation.) The tests you will see most frequently mentioned in published research papers are Pearson's product movement, Spearman's rho and Kendall's tau. (The reader is referred to the Bibliography for further suggested reading on statistical analyses.)

3 More complex analysis of a number of sets of scores examining the extent to which they vary together. For instance, you might want to know about the effects of different treatments on a group of patients, taking into account their age and sex.

Analysis of variance (Anova) is a more complex analysis because it can cope with a number of different sets of scores and their interactions. You will certainly need skilled help if this method is to be used. Although these tests can be performed by hand it is a very time consuming task and computers are usually used. The packages most commonly used are:

SPSS Statistical Package for the Social Sciences. Norusis M. J. McGraw-Hill, New York

BMDP Biomedical Data Package (1981). University of California, California.

These notes only give a broad idea of the tests; in order to use them each test makes certain assumptions about the data to be analysed, which is why expert advice is needed.

It is useful to remember that there are two broad categories of statistical tests: parametric and non-parametric. *Parametric tests* are suitable for use with data which are normally distributed and with data obtained from ratio scales. The normal distribution is often mentioned and is based on the statistical notion of a normal curve.

A normal curve looks bell-shaped and is shown in Figure 10.4. It is based on the assumption that if enough data are collected about a particular characteristic most people will have a value in the middle of the range, while a few people will fall at the extremes. Height is a good illustration. In a gathering of 100 people there are likely to be a few people over 1.8 m (6 feet) tall and a similar number below 1.5 m (5 feet), but the majority will be in between. A possible distribution curve is given in Figure 10.5.

The reader is advised to refer to some of the statistics books given in the Bibliography for further information about normal distributions.

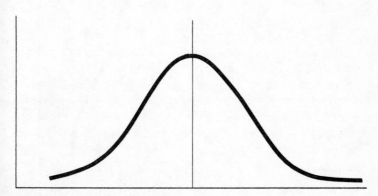

Fig. 10.4   *Normal distribution curve.*

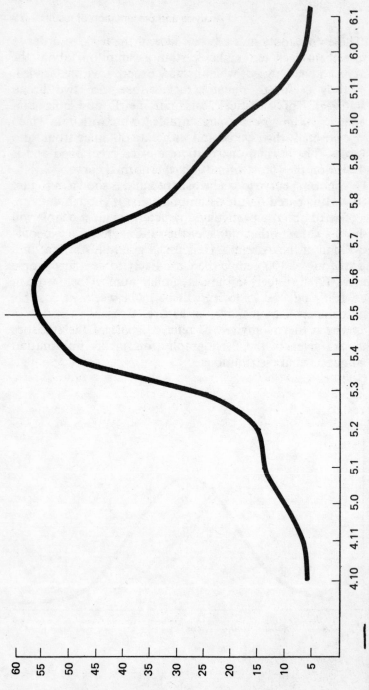

Fig. 10.5 Distribution of height of members attending an international conference

If the population does not follow a normal distribution it is said to be skewed (Fig. 10.6).

Using the example of height of people attending a conference (Fig. 10.15), the curve is 'skewed' towards the left and therefore indicates more small people in this sample—although the range is the same.

Non-parametric tests do not make assumptions about the normal distribution of the data and can cope with nominal and ordinal scale values. However, non-parametric tests require substantial differences between sets of scores before significance in the results can be obtained.

When you have information from open questions as discussed in Chapter 8, where you have asked a general question such as 'How do you feel about your accident?' or 'In what ways has your life been affected by your present illness?', it is not possible to list the answers in the same way as with closed questions and the method of *content analysis* is frequently used. This method is a highly developed special purpose technique mainly developed for use in political science, psychology and social anthropology, but which can be adapted for use by any discipline wishing to examine written material. The aim of the analysis is to improve the quality of the inferences made about what is recorded. Material in research may be collected in written form or tape recorded and later transcribed. Content

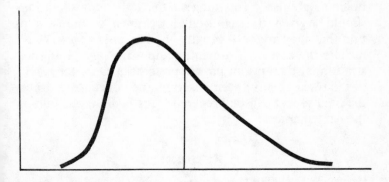

Fig. 10.6   *Skewed curve.*

analysis provides a means of being objective and systematic about this material. Without this systematic investigation, personal bias will tend to influence what is extracted. For example, a researcher trying to obtain evidence for a particular point of view is more likely to pick up evidence supporting this hypothesis than statements which contradict it. The technique of content analysis can be mastered by anyone prepared to spend the time on learning. The reader is referred to Carney (1972) for further detailed information.

Whatever method is adopted for handling and analysing the data a clear picture of the information must be retained and how this relates to the original research question.

Sophisticated computer printouts and numerous results of statistical tests will mean nothing unless interpreted by the researcher with in-depth knowledge of the project. Any significant relationships found will need to be interpreted within the context of the project and discussed in relation to the research question, the hypotheses proposed, and objectives set.

When results are not found to be statistically significant discussion is still needed. Non-significant results can be important for practice. Suppose that a piece of research has been carried out to compare two treatments, A and B, and the researcher finds that there are no significant differences between the two treatments when several measures of outcome are used. This suggests that other considerations should be given to selecting either treatment on the assumption that they are both equally good or poor. These could include the cost of treatment, equipment, ease of administration, or therapist or patient preference. Once the results of the research have been analysed and conclusions drawn the final report can be prepared. This is discussed fully in the next chapter.

References

Carney T. F. (1972). *Content Analysis*. Manitoba: University of Manitoba Press.

Graham W. G. B., Bradley D. A. (1978). Efficacy of chest physiotherapy and intermittent positive pressure breathing in the resolution of pneumonia. *New England Journal of Medicine*, **229,** 624–627.

11 Writing the Research Report and Publicising the Results

The research report

For most people, writing is a time consuming task, and research reports present particular difficulties. Because there is a conventional way of presenting research material, your report should follow the recognised format, which is standardised in a logical way to make it easier for others to read and understand. The order given here is that in which the report should be presented, but is probably not the order in which you actually write it; summaries and introductions in particular are usually easier to write after other sections have been completed.

Most people find the best way to approach the task is to write a section, put it firmly away for a week or so, and then come back to it. Many grammatical and other errors will be immediately obvious and you can then correct them. If you try to correct too soon after you have written the section, mistakes are more difficult to see. It is also helpful to ask at least one other person to read and comment on drafts of the report. You need comments on the actual content from someone knowledgeable about your topic, and criticism of style and layout, the latter possibly from a different source. It is often helpful to read a few reports by other experienced researchers before you start writing your own. The headings under which the report should be presented are as follows.

Title

This is important as it should attract attention to your work in the first place. It must be accurate and not too long. A few examples may help:

> Practicalities of achieving collaboration between hospital and community-based services in the care of the elderly mentally infirm.
>
> Rather offputting!
>
> Community services for the elderly mentally infirm: cooperation or competition?
>
> Simpler and more to the point.

> The outcome of patients with a nailed hip fracture requiring rehabilitation in a hospital for chronic care.
>
> A little long—perhaps too much detail.
>
> Rehabilitation outcomes following a fractured hip.
>
> Simpler, more likely to arouse interest.

Often by the time you get to the end of a research project the original title is no longer appropriate—if this is so, change it and possibly explain why you have done so if your original title has already been publicised.

Summary

This should contain a brief analytical outline of the problem and the background to the study, the objectives or the hypotheses proposed, the methods used in the investigation, and the results obtained. About 100 words is a suitable length. Summaries are surprisingly difficult to write and here many rewrites may be necessary. It is essential that this section is clear and concise; if it is not, the reader may go no further!

Introduction

This sets the scene for the whole study, gives some background information with reference to other work in the area, and clearly defines the purpose of the study.

General expectations about the outcome of the investigation should be mentioned, with some of the reasons on which they are based. In your discussion section you will refer back to points raised here in the introduction, and the extent to which expectations were fulfilled or reasons why they were not.

Methods

The first part describes the general features of the approach and the research design used, i.e. whether it was a survey, descriptive study or clinical trial. Details that are appropriate will vary with the type of study but some information about the study population and how it was selected is essential, with criteria for inclusion and exclusion if these are used; the reader needs to be reassured that bias in selection was avoided.

The procedure followed must be clearly described—the guiding principle here is that there should be sufficient detail for someone else to replicate the study. If the method used is a well-recognised one or an adaptation of a well-known one, then reference can be made to the original work, but with mention of attempts to check appropriateness of methods for use with your study population. If tools of measurement have been developed particularly for the study, details of development work and of the extent of validity for the purpose and reliability in use should be given.

Full details of questionnaires and other forms used are given in the Appendix, but examples of some of the questions can be given here to give the flavour of the study.

It is often difficult to decide what to include in this section and what to put in the Appendix. The answer is to write up this section in full, then later decide what would be better placed elsewhere in the interests of clarity and easy reading.

One of the problems in writing this type of report is making sure that under each heading information that belongs there—and only that—is given. It is very easy to find results creeping in before you actually come to that section. For example in the methods section when describing a questionnaire it is tempting to add 'the response rate was 80%'. You may be very proud of this, but it must wait until the results section. Remember to check for this kind of error, which can be annoying for the reader and also means that the results section has less impact. The whole report should follow through logically from the reasons for setting up the study, what you proposed to do, how you did it, and on to what you found.

Results

This is another section which easily gets mixed up with the following one—discussion. The results section should contain only *facts*, not discussion or opinion. Clear *summaries* of the data in form of tables, graphs, etc., are appropriate—full details of calculation and raw data are given in the Appendix. Remember that all tables and graphs must be clearly labelled and comprehensible on their own without reference to the text. Check that if abbreviations are used, e.g. FTE (full-time equivalent), the full wording is also given nearby, also check that each axis is labelled on graphs, and each table is numbered and has a heading. Data need only be presented in one form, e.g. if a summary table is given, it is not necessary to also give these results fully in the text.

Discussion

Some interpretation of the results is needed here, including the remarks that crept into the results section. The findings should be considered in relation to previous work, in the same or related areas. Also discussion of the results in relation to problems specified in the introduction, and the extent to which expectations were realised, and if not why not. Real life research rarely works out as you expect for many different reasons. Results rarely 'prove' anything: they may support hypotheses or other work but the term *proof* is not appropriate as knowledge is always advancing. What you 'prove' today may, with new knowledge, be 'disproved' tomorrow.

In any research a full report of all the findings should be written up and funding bodies will normally require this. This full report is the only evidence you have of all your hard work, it also provides material for talks, lectures and written papers. Reports are not often published in full, so it is important to publicise your findings in other ways. Each journal has its own format—and may have rules about ways in which articles may be presented. It is worthwhile paying a lot of attention to this as good material may be turned down because its style or presentation is not suitable for the journal.

Conclusion

A brief restatement of findings and the implications of them is given here. It requires practice not to be merely repetitive, rewriting (and rewriting) is often the only way to solve the problem.

References

References to articles and books which you have mentioned throughout the text of the report must be listed at the end. There are a number of different systems, but what is essential is consistency, all written in the same way even down to the punctuation. References can either be numbered chronologically throughout the text and listed by number at the end, or names given with dates in the text and listed alphabetically according to the name of the first author in the reference section. Which you decide to do may depend on the number of references you have used. What is most important here is that anyone wishing to obtain the papers or books you refer to has sufficient detail to be able to do so.

Examples of references:
Harvard system:
Journal reference

> Wall P. (1985). The discovery of transcutaneous electrical nerve stimulation. *Physiotherapy*, **71**, (8) 348–350.
> Black K. D., Halverson J. L., Majerus K. A., Soderburg G. L. (1985). Alterations in ankle dorsiflexion torque as a result of continuous ultrasound to the anterior tibial compartment. *Physical Therapy*, **64**, (6), 910–918.

Book reference

> Levin H. M. (1985). *Cost-effectiveness: A Primer*. Beverley Hills: Sage Publications.

Chapter in book:

> Lee P. R., Franks P. E. (1980). Health and disease in the community. In *Primary Care* (Fry J. P., ed.) pp. 3–34. London: William Heinemann Medical Books.

Publicising your results

It is extremely important you make sure that as many people as possible know about the results of your study. This is done in two main ways: by giving talks and by writing papers. Unfortunately each will have to be done separately—a written paper is unsuitable for verbal presentation and vice versa.

Talking at meetings

It is a good idea when you are nearing the end of your study to consider where you might present a paper about it. Many societies and conferences are keen to encourage prospective speakers. Consider your audience and slant your talk so that it will be of maximum interest to them. For example, a therapist talking to a therapist audience may stress details of treatment techniques used and detailed implications of the results for practice. To a wider audience, you might want to include financial and management implications, and perhaps for a medical audience, how these particular results have implications for the wider overall management of this diagnostic group.

Well-prepared visual aids, and rehearsal, will help to ensure good presentation. Educational psychologists have said if you want your message to have an impact only introduce one new idea every three minutes. Repetition of the same idea in different ways is essential in a talk. If it is only one idea in three minutes, you can only introduce three or four in a ten-minute paper. Even if you have only ten minutes, set the scene of your paper for your audience so that they are ready to receive the information about your results. For example: 'There has been an interest in monitoring gait for many years both among clinicians and biomedical engineers but evidence of collaborative work is sadly lacking...' You go on to tell of the marvellous research that has been achieved in your work with biomedical engineers!

Writing a paper

The paper that you want to publish is quite different from the talk. Your speaking style may be fairly informal with the use of 'I' and 'we', you will repeat points for emphasis and few references will be given. Writing style will be formal, usually past tense third person, and there should be no repetition. Papers will also contain much less information than your final report. A large report may generate a number of different papers.

The first step when considering publication is to read journals that might be appropriate, to find out about their layout and the general style of articles. There is a very wide variation in different journals and your article will only be considered if it fits in with the journal's general style and interests. Most journals also give guidelines as to the style they require.

Most professions have their own journals but it is also a good idea to consider going to a wider audience as well: would other professions be interested in your results? Would it be helpful if they were?

Sometimes when you reach the end of your research and have written the report, you are heartily sick of the whole topic. Leave it for a month or so and then come back to consider papers and talks.

12 Notes on Critical Appraisal of a Research Report

There are many different ways of considering a research report, and those who are unfamiliar with the layout or presentation may find it difficult to judge the value of a particular paper and decide the weight that should be given to the findings. A few guidelines may be helpful in identifying some of the things to look for.

A research article should be about facts, a well written article should be easy to read and understand—the use of jargon or obscure phraseology often intended to impress, usually only confuses. Stephen Lock in *Better Medical Writing* (1977) includes the following among his list of 'pseud' words that are pompous and often meaningless in the context in which they are used: normative, meaningful, seminal, multidisciplinary, statementise. Good, clear English needs time. A number of questions have been asked here which help to highlight different aspects of a research report.

Importance, relevance and definition

Is the topic important, is the research question a reasonable one and has it been clearly defined? If the answer to all three is not in the affirmative, maybe there is no point in going further. If the topic is important but the question irrelevant, the findings are of little interest.

What is the background to the study?

There should be enough information in the introduction to set the scene, and to identify the purpose of the study. The authors may want to challenge previous work, or fill gaps in existing work in the area.

How did they do it?

The importance of any results and the reliance that can be placed on them must depend on the methods used.

1 Are they clearly described and were they appropriate?
2 Is evidence of the reliability and validity of any tools of measurement used given?
3 How were the subjects of the study selected? Have attempts been made to obtain a representative sample?
4 If any treatment was part of the study, was this clearly defined? Exactly what was done and by whom? If treatments are standardised for the purposes of the study, do these standard treatments still make sense in terms of patient care? In the following example treatments are standardised to the extent that they in no way reflect actual practice.

Treatment was standardised as follows:

1 Breathing exercises: five lateral costal breaths and five diaphragmatic breaths.
2 Postural drainage given to all patients in prone, supine and both lateral positions three minutes in each position (Newton and Stephenson, 1978).

---

5 If outcome measures are used in an evaluative study, do these really relate to the treatment? Two outcome measures frequently reported are the use of pain-killing drugs, and return to work. Either of these used on their own may tell little about the effects of treatment: the use of pain-killing drugs may have more to do with ward routines, or the patient 'finishing off the tablets' than actual changes in pain; and time off work is notoriously influenced by a large number of factors, including the type of job in relation to the problem, the extent to which the individual finds the job satisfying or not, or financial rewards and losses—self-employed people normally return to work much quicker than those in the employ of others.

6 The number of subjects is important, it is not possible to generalise when only small numbers are used, although in-depth studies often use small numbers and provide a basis for further study. Big is not always beautiful, and wise authors who use small numbers draw attention to this and do not claim to be able to generalise; i.e. results of work done with 20 patients should not form on its own a basis for a recommendation for change.

What did they find?

Are the results clearly presented? Are the methods of analysis appropriate—if only small numbers are used, is complex statistical analysis justified? Beware when percentages are much larger than actual figures, i.e. $4 = 25\%$—reminiscent of the report of a study of mice—one-third recovered following treatment, one-third died and ... the other one got away!

Statistical analysis should be used to clarify, not to mystify. Remember that statistical significance does not necessarily mean real-life significance, e.g. although the test shows the increase in range of movement is statistically significant, functionally the patient may be no better off, therefore the increase has no real-life significance.

Here it should be mentioned how to interpret the $P < 0.05$ or $P < 0.01$ which frequently occurs at the bottom of a statistical calculation. This refers to 'probabilities', and means that as a result of performing some test on the data the result obtained would only have been obtained by chance five times out of 100 (0.05) or once in every 100 (0.01). If the significance is even greater it may be given as 0.001, in which case only once in a thousand times would this result have occurred by chance.

Discussion and recommendations

Do these really relate to the study, are the author's claims justified by his data? Personal opinion often creeps in and suggestions made are not based on the data of the study. It is worth checking on this.

When you find a recommendation for action go back to the paper and see if it is based on reported findings or not. If not it will probably reflect the author's opinion. Separating fact from opinion is one of the most important tasks in reading a research paper.

Other points it may be worth considering

Does the paper read well? Even complex material well presented should be understandable. Is there good use of visual material—clearly labelled tables, figures and diagrams. Do remember that if you have to spend a long time puzzling over a table or figure trying to understand it, then probably it is the table that is at fault, not your intelligence!

If you are evaluating a paper you often feel intuitively that it is not a good one, but it is necessary to sort out exactly why. These suggestions may be helpful to start with. The habit of reading research articles and discussing them with others will help to develop a standard against which to consider new articles and it will become easier and more interesting.

Specific questions must be asked about the paper so that particular aspects can be considered. This is much more helpful than considering them as a whole. An interesting research project may be badly written up and one that reads well may have little to contribute.

To make the best use of reading the research and acquiring the skill of critical appraisal, make notes when you read a scientific article, and underline or use a coloured pen to highlight important points. Journal clubs are an excellent means of helping to develop critical skills in a group.

References

Lock S. (1977). *Thorne's Better Medical Writing*, 2nd edn. London: Pitman Medical.

Newton D. A. G., Stephenson A. (1978). Effect of physiotherapy on pulmonary function: a laboratory study. *Lancet*, **2**, 228–230.

Glossary

This section gives the meanings of a number of terms used in research; it is useful to remember that some may have other meanings when used in other situations.

Averages (measures of central tendency)

Mean

Most people think of the mean as the average. It is calculated by dividing the total sum of the items by the number of the items involved.

$8 + 7 + 4 + 2 + 6 + 4 + 3 + 4 + 9 = 47$

$47 \div 9 = \underline{5.22}$ This is the mean.

Mode

This together with the mean and the following median show how scores are grouped. The mode is the item that occurs most frequently—in the above example the mode is *4*.

Median

This is simply the middle item of a set of scores. Arrange the scores in order from smallest to largest and the middle one in the array is the median. Using the above example:

2,3,4,4,$\underline{4}$,6,7,8,9, the fifth item, which is in the middle of 9 is 4—the median. If there are an even number of items in an array take the mean of the two middle numbers as the median, add them together and divide by 2.

e.g. 2,3,4,4,$\underline{4,5}$,6,7,8,9

    $4 + 5 = 9$

    $9 \div 2 = \underline{4.5}$

Correlation

When scores on two factors are correlated it means that they covary in some way. A positive correlation means that when one goes up or down, the other moves in the same direction, a negative correlation means that when one rises the other falls. For example, there is usually a positive correlation in children between chronological age and reading ability. There might be a negative correlation between speed of handwriting and legibility.

Causality

This is often confused with correlation above. Because two items covary it does not mean that one causes the other. There may be a third factor which influences both. The example often quoted which illustrates this well is in the United States Economic Statistics: clergymen's salaries are shown to correlate with liquor sales. The assumption could be made that when vicars' salaries increased they bought more liquor, but this would be incorrect because further investigation of the figures shows that the general financial climate was affecting both salaries and liquor sales. In research, causality can only be demonstrated in strictly controlled experimental investigations.

Controlled trial

This can mean two things: either a trial which is appropriately scientific and therefore to that extent controlled; or a trial in which there is a 'control' group, i.e. one which is receiving no active treatment and with which the other treatment groups can be compared.

Data

These are the actual figures, statements or other information you obtain. Raw data are the figures before any analysis is done. It is often forgotten that it is a plural noun. Datum is the singular.

Ethics

This refers to moral issues; what is morally correct and honourable. Ethical issues are discussed in Chapter 7.

Incidence/prevalence

These mean slightly different things and are epidemiological terms. Incidence refers to the actual frequency of occurrence of something—for example, the number of new strokes that occurred within the population at risk within a specified health district. Prevalence is the total number of persons with a disease or other characteristic in a defined population. Prevalence can be expressed as point prevalence; that is, at any given point in time or over any specified period of time such as a year or a month.

International classification of disease (ICD)

This is a classification of all diseases into numbered categories and sub-categories. Two books are available which are updated from time to time by the World Health Organisation in Geneva. By using this method disease categories are understood world-wide—it helps to some extent to deal with the different diagnostic terms sometimes used for the same condition.

Objective

The term objective refers to that which can be shown to be independent of any bias, by its nature it is not affected by observers' thoughts or feelings. If a distance walked is to be measured then a measured walkway must be used or a milometer attached to the patient; several independent observers watching the patient will agree on the distance walked because it is objectively measured.

Parameter

The dictionary definition of this word is 'quantity constant in case considered but varying in different cases'—it derives from the Greek word to measure. It is used in research to denote the variables you are selecting to measure a particular property. For example, you may decide to use the time taken to walk a measured distance as a measure of walking ability, or performance of self-care tasks as a measure of dressing ability.

Protocol

Another word for the research proposal or the formal plan you have worked out for your study.

Random allocation or random selection

If patients or subjects are to be included in your study or divided into groups, it must be clear that any selection or allocation is free from bias and is really random. This does not mean haphazard, it means you have used a system that eliminates any possible bias. If there was no set system, those who you think are going to do well might be more likely to be allocated to the active treatment group. The conditions for selection must be stated in advance and then strictly adhered to. There are many different ways this can be done: by the use of a random numbers table, a pre-arranged system of cards or even picking names out of a hat!

Random numbers

Tables of random numbers can be found at the back of some books on statistics, they can also be generated by using a computer. They are used in random allocation (*see above*).

Range

This is the range covered by your scores and is shown by giving the lowest and highest scores in your sample, e.g. range 18–33, 18 the lowest score obtained, 33 the highest.

Reliability

This can refer to three main aspects:

1 Do different people using the test to measure the same thing obtain the same scores?
2 Does the same person on different occasions obtain the same scores?
3 On re-testing in a situation where nothing is expected to have changed are similar scores obtained?

A problem here in remedial therapy is that often it is recovery and change that are being monitored and therefore change over time may reflect actual change, rather than unreliability of the test; this must be considered.

Repeatability

This is used in relation to methods of measurement and refers to the extent to which the same measurement can be obtained using the same instrument on different occasions — if the property being measured is still the same. Test, re-test methods examine the extent of repeatability of a test.

Response set

This is something to be avoided. It means that when setting out a questionnaire the questions should not be set out in such a way that the respondent can always put yes in the same place. People may answer 'yes' to the first four questions and become 'set' in that method of answering. Phrase questions so that people have to think about answering them.

For example:

In a rating scale do not have either right or left hand consistently representing one aspect.

Good .... Bad
Pleasant .... Unpleasant

rather

Good .... Bad
Unpleasant .... Pleasant

This helps to ensure that respondents give due weight to each question individually.

Sample

Refers to the population or group you select for your study.

Sample size

Refers to the size of the population that is being studied.

Scales

Scales of measurement can be of different kinds, those most frequently found are nominal, ordinal, interval, and ratio scales. It is important to consider which sort of scale you are using as this will decide the kind of analysis that is appropriate, and the interpretations you can make from your data. The four types of scales are explained below with examples.

Nominal

In this type of scale things or people are assigned to groups on the basis of nominal differences for example, brands of Scotch whisky can be assorted according to brand names, one brand is no more 'Scotch' than another, merely different. In health care, the terms 'unaffected' and 'affected' are often used. These are nominal classifications. For example, in a patient with a fractured femur, we refer to the affected and unaffected leg, while for stroke patients the division may be into those with sensory or perceptual problems, and those without. These categories are extremely broad and though they may be useful for descriptive purposes, no further assumptions can be made from this type of classification, i.e. about the type of fracture or the extent of sensory or perceptual problems. Though you may choose to assign numbers to these groups they mean nothing.

Ordinal measurement

This type of scale can be very useful in monitoring and assessing different aspects of patient care. It means that an order can be imposed on certain items but that the interval between these items has no numerical significance. A good example of this in everyday life is military rank. A corporal, as a rank, is not only different from a private in the nominal sense but higher. If you assign the number 1 to a private, 2 to a corporal and 3 to a sergeant these numbers have ordinal properties, both 2 and 3 are higher than 1; however, the interval between the numbers does not have any particular significance, 2 privates do not equal one corporal! Ranking scales are used to measure such things as pain, or patient satisfaction.

Interval measurement

An example of an interval scale is Celsius temperature scale where the difference say between 25° and 50° is the same as that between 50° and 75°. The intervals are meaningful but the numbers themselves are not because on this scale 0 does not represent zero, it is only a convenient reference point—the freezing point of water. This type of scale does not have much application in remedial therapy, although a dolorimeter looking like a thermometer is sometimes used to measure pain.

Ratio measurement

The classic ratio scales are length, mass and time. Here one can make assumptions which are not valid in the other scales; that 10 cm is twice as long as 5 cm, that 10 minutes is half as long as 20 minutes, that 12 paces are twice as many as 6. With these scales many forms of statistical analysis, not justified in the other scales, can be used. Although these scales are clearly the most rigorous type of measurement and give the most information, what is most important when selecting a scale is that it is appropriate for the purpose. Doctors and others examining remedial therapy from the outside sometimes use tests which of themselves appear very robust but are quite inappropriate for measuring the property being investigated.

Standard deviation (SD)

This is a measure of dispersion that shows how your scores are distributed around the mean. You will often find that the mean, range and standard deviation of scores are given. There is a simple formula for calculating the standard deviation and the reader is again referred to the statistical books suggested in the Bibliography.

Statistics

Numerical information systematically collected, is the dictionary definition. Statistics are really the figures or numbers you collect.

Statistical analysis

This refers to the tests which are used to examine the data to find out about differences and similarities. Statistical analysis is used on the data you have collected to test the hypotheses you have proposed.

Subjective

The meaning of this term is frequently misunderstood and viewed with suspicion, but subjective data can form an important source of information. It concerns individual feelings, opinions, and attitudes. We may want to know a patient's opinions about his progress, his feelings about what has happened, or his opinions about the treatment he has received. Where problems arise is when these subjective data are regarded as objective, i.e. the doctor's or therapist's opinion about the patient's progress is regarded as 'evidence' of that progress or lack of it, rather than as opinions about progress.

Subjects

This refers to the people (or it could be animals) included in your study. They become subjects when you start studying them.

Validity

This is a term often used in relation to tests and other tools of measurement. It has many aspects though people tend to just report 'the test was valid'. The following are ways in which a test may be considered in terms of validity.

Face validity

This refers to what the test appears to measure—whether it 'looks' valid and concerns the public relations aspect. Does the test appear to relate directly to the purpose that has been explained to the participants?

Criterion related

This refers to the extent to which the test compares with others claiming to measure similar items, and how it works practically in a test situation. For example, if you are examining a test claiming to measure disability, how does it compare with other tests of disability? If used with a population of disabled patients, do those more severely disabled obtain scores that are different from those less disabled? Does it discriminate between those who are disabled and those who are not?

Construct related

This refers to the extent to which the test measures the underlying construct or trait. For example, if a test is of disability in everyday life, to what extent do the items actually relate to this? Many tests may only relate to performance in a particular situation and not real-life situations of performance of activities. The correlations between scores on the test you are examining and others should not be too high, otherwise your test may just be duplicating others; however, the length or ease of administration could be a reason for choosing it.

Content validity

Do the items in the test cover a representative sample of the behaviour that is to be measured? For example, if the test is of functional ability of a specified area, say hand function, does it reasonably cover most aspects of hand function?

Variables

This is the term used in experimental investigations for properties that are being studied and which can vary. Common examples are age, sex, height, intelligence, performance of movements and activities, social or economic status. Some variables such as sex are mutually exclusive, e.g. if you are male you cannot also be female (except in the rarest circumstances). Other variables, such as height, can be measured along a continuum. The terms independent and dependent variable are also used.

Independent variable

This is the term used in an investigation for the variables you are manipulating, the treatments you are giving or the interventions you are introducing, for example, independent variables could be a specific treatment, an orthosis, length of time on treatment, age or severity of condition. You are interested in the effect of these variables on the dependent variable.

Dependent variable

This is the property you are using as your 'outcome'. You may want to examine the effect of a regimen of exercise on walking ability or a programme of training on voice production. In these examples walking ability and voice production are the dependent variables, the regimen of exercise and the programme of training are the independent variables. In this kind of investigation you are examining the effect of the independent variables on the dependent variable.

Bibliography

Berry R. (1978). *How to Write a Research Paper*. Oxford: Pergamon Press.

Beveridge W. I. B. (1974). *The Art of Scientific Investigation*. London: Heinemann Educational Books.

Blalock H. M. (1970). *An Introduction to Social Research*. Maidenhead: Prentice Hall.

Borchardt D. H., Francis R. D. (1984). *How to Find Out in Psychology: A Guide to the Literature and Methods of Research*. Oxford: Pergamon Press.

Borg W. R., Gall M. D. (1979). *Educational Research—An Introduction*, 3rd edn. New York: Longmans.

Bradford Hill A. (1979). *Medical Statistics*. London: Hodder and Stoughton.

Broughton Pipkin F. (1984). *Medical Statistics Made Easy*. London: Churchill Livingstone.

Buros O. K. (1974). *Tests in Print II, A Master Index for Seven Mental Measurement Year Books*. New Jersey: Gryphon Press.

Buros O. K. (1975). *Tests in Print III*. New Jersey: Gryphon Press.

Bynner J., Stribley R. (1979). *Social Research, Principles and Procedures*. London: Longmans.

Calnan J. (1976). *One Way to do Research*. London: William Heinemann Medical Books.

Clarke D. H., Clarke H. H. (1970). *Research Processes in Physical Education, Recreation and Health*. Englewood Cliffs, New Jersey: Prentice Hall Inc.

Cromwell L., Weibell F. J., Pfeiffer E. A. *et al.* (1973). *Biomedical Instrumentation and Measurements*. Englewood Cliffs, New Jersey: Prentice Hall Inc.

Evans K. M. (1968). *Planning Small Scale Research*. Windsor, Berks: National Foundation for Educational Research.

Gowers E. (1964). *The Complete Plain Words*. London: HMSO.

Hersen M., Barlow D. H. (1976). *Single Case Experimental Design*. Oxford: Pergamon Press.

Huff D. (1978). *How to Lie with Statistics*. London: Pelican.

Jantzen A. C. (1981). *Research: The Practical Approach for Occupational Therapy*. Maryland: RAMSCO Laurel.

Krausz E., Miller S. H. (1978). *Social Research Design*. London: Longmans.

Lock S. (1977). *Thorne's Better Medical Writing*, 2nd edn. London: Pitman Medical.

Moroney M. J. (1978). *Facts from Figures*. London: Pelican.

Moser C. A., Kalton G. (1978). *Survey Methods in Social Investigation*. London: Heinemann Educational Books Limited.

Oppenheim A. N. (1982). *Questionnaire Design and Attitude Measurement*. London: Heinemann Educational Books.

Phillips D. S. (1978). *Basic Statistics for Health Science Students*. San Francisco: Freeman and Company.

✗ Robson C. (1979). *Experiment, Design and Statistics in Psychology*. Harmondsworth: Penguin Books Limited.

Sainsbury S. (1973). *Measuring Disability*. London: Bell.

Shepherd M. (ed.) (1984). *Spectrum of Psychiatric Research*. Cambridge: Cambridge University Press.

Shouksmith G. (1978). *Assessment through Interviewing*, 2nd edn. Oxford: Pergamon International Library.

Siegel S. (1956). *Non-parametric Statistics for the Behavioural Sciences*. London: McGraw-Hill.

Simon J. L. (1978). *Basic Research Methods in Social Science*, 2nd edn. New York: Random House Inc.

Stacey M. (1969). *Methods of Social Research*. Oxford: Pergamon Press.

Treece E. W., Treece J. W. (1977). *Elements of Research in Nursing*, 2nd edn. St Louis: Mosby and Company.

Willis L. D., Linwood M. E. (1984). *Measuring the Quality of Care*. Edinburgh: Churchill Livingstone.

Wilson M. (ed.) (1979). *Social and Educational Research in Action. A Book of Readings*. London: Longmans.

Witt P. (1980). *Research Writing Tips*. Alexandria, Virginia: American Physical Therapy Association.

Yeoman K. A. (1968). *Statistics for the Social Scientist, Vols. I and II*. Harmondsworth: Penguin Education.

Index